Positive Options for Crohn's Disease

Dr. Joan Gomez is Honorary Consulting Psychiatrist to the Chelsea and Westminster Hospital. She was trained at King's College, London, and Westminster Hospital, and obtained her Diploma in Psychological Medicine and Membership of the Royal College of Psychiatry in 1973 and 1974 respectively. She was elected a Fellow of the Royal College of Psychiatrists in 1982, and obtained the Diploma in the History of Medicine in 1996 and the Diploma in the Philosophy of Medicine in 1998. She is a Fellow of the Society of Apothecaries and also of the Royal Society of Medicine. She has been engaged in clinical work and research on the interface between psychiatry and physical medicine. Dr. Gomez is also the author of four other books: *Coping with Thyroid Problems* (1994), *How to Cope with Bulimia* (1995), *Living with Diabetes* (1995), and *How to Cope with Anemia* (1998).

FOR MY CAT, EMMA, A DELIGHTFUL COMPANION

Ordering

Trade bookstores in the U.S. and Canada please contact:

Publishers Group West
1700 Fourth Street, Berkeley CA 94710
Phone: (800) 788-3123
Fax: (510) 528-3444

Hunter House books are available at bulk discounts for textbook course adoptions; to qualifying community, healthcare, and government organizations; and for special promotions and fundraising. For details please contact:

Special Sales Department
Hunter House Inc., PO Box 2914, Alameda CA 94501-0914
Tel. (510) 865-5282   Fax (510) 865-4295
e-mail: ordering@hunterhouse.com

Individuals can order our books from most bookstores or by calling toll-free:
1-800-266-5592

Positive Options

FOR

CROHN'S

DISEASE

Self-Help and Treatment

Joan Gomez, M.D.

Hunter House Inc., Publishers
P.O. Box 2914
Alameda CA 94501-0914

First published in Great Britain in 2000 by
Sheldon Press, SPCK, Marylebone Road, London NW1 4DU

Library of Congress Cataloging-in-Publication Data

Gomez, Joan.
    Positive options for Crohn's disease : self-help and treatment /
Joan Gomez.—1st ed.
        p. cm.
    Includes index.
    ISBN 0-89793-278-1 (paper)   ISBN 0-89793-279-X (cloth)
    1. Enteritis, Regional—Popular works. I. Title.
    RC862.E52 G66 2000
    616.3'445—dc21   00-021084

Project credits
Cover Design: Brian Dittmar Graphic Design
Book Production: Hunter House
Copy Editor: Kelley Blewster
Proofreader: Lee Rappold
Indexer: Kathy Talley-Jones
Production Director: Virginia Fontana
Acquisitions Coordinator: Jeanne Brondino
Associate Editor: Alex Mummery
Publicity Director: Marisa Spatafore
Sales Coordinator: Sarah Kulin
Customer Service Manager: Christina Sverdrup
Order fulfillment: Joel Irons, A & A Quality Shipping Services

Printed and Bound by Bang Printing, Brainerd, Minnesota
Manufactured in the United States of America

9 8 7 6 5 4   First Edition   04 05 06 07

Contents

Important Note

The material in this book is intended to provide a review of resources and information related to Crohn's Disease. Every effort has been made to provide accurate and dependable information. However, professionals in the field may have differing opinions and change is always taking place. Any of the treatments described herein should be undertaken only under the guidance of a licensed health care practitioner. The author, editors, and publishers cannot be held responsible for any error, omission, professional disagreement, outdated material, or adverse outcomes that derive from use of any of these treatments or information resources in this book, either in a program of self-care or under the care of a licensed practitioner.

What Crohn's Disease Is and Why It Matters

Crohn's is essentially a disease of civilization—our own modern Western variety—and it is increasing alarmingly. By 1994 Professor Hermon-Taylor of St. George's Hospital, London, was calling it an epidemic. It used to be a rarity and did not even have a name until the 1930s. It is still rare in the developing countries, although becoming less so as they "catch" our lifestyle. It is particularly prevalent in the cities of North America, Western Europe, and Australia. It is well known in New York, London, Sydney, or Copenhagen, but not so common in sparsely populated rural areas such as Iceland and northern Norway.

HOW CROHN'S DISEASE WAS DISCOVERED

Although Crohn's disease acquired its name and identity only 70 years ago, as far back as 600 B.C. the Greek physician Asklepios was treating patients with bowel disorders. In his open-air health clinic he prescribed a regimen of fasting, diet, rest, and "healing dreams" (something like hypnosis). We would find his treatment perfectly acceptable today. After the Greeks, hundreds of years went by without any significant medical advances.

Much later, in 1769, Giovanni Morgagni described a young man suffering from a chronic, debilitating illness with diarrhea, which we might recognize today as Crohn's disease. At about the

1

same time, Bonnie Prince Charlie complained of a persistent "bloody flux"—this could have been the same problem. He cured himself by cutting out dairy products—a treatment still used today. In fact, in 1996 it was suggested by one group of doctors that mycobacteria in milk were the cause of the disease. In 1905, Dr. Heinrich Albert Johne, in Germany, discovered a disease of the intestines in cattle that is very like Crohn's disease—but at that time no one had recognized the human version.

Dr. Samuel Wilks of Guy's Hospital set the ball rolling in 1859 by writing and lecturing about his patient, Isabella Bankes, a recognizable—to us—Crohn's disease sufferer. Other colleagues became interested. In 1913, Dr. Dalziel of Glasgow described a whole group of similar patients suffering from what was still an illness without a name.

In 1930 Dr. Burrill Crohn came on the scene. He was working at the Mount Sinai Hospital in New York and was at his wits' end over a 17-year-old patient. The boy had a high temperature, pain in the abdomen, diarrhea, and a tender lump in the appendix area. Dr. Crohn suspected a tuberculous infection, but the youngster did not respond to the existing treatment. A dangerous operation was the only way to find out what was wrong, but the situation became desperate and Dr. Crohn's colleague, Dr. A. A. Berg, decided to take the risk.

The lump turned out to be a hard mass of inflamed tissue at the lower end of the small intestine, the ileum. The big question was, what caused the inflammation? Even today, although we have plenty of theories, we are still not sure. By 1932 Dr. Crohn had researched several more cases and presented a paper about this "new" illness at a meeting of the American Medical Association in New Orleans. He called it *regional ileitis*—inflammation of the ileum, usually affecting the last section. (Classical or typical Crohn's disease is an inflammation of the ileum.) During the 1960s it became clear that the characteristic patches of inflammation, causing fever and diarrhea, could crop up anywhere in the digestive tract, and the name *Crohn's disease* came to be used instead.

INFLAMMATORY BOWEL DISEASE (IBD)

Inflammatory bowel disease—not to be confused with IBS, the common irritable bowel syndrome—is an umbrella term doctors use for Crohn's disease and another illness called ulcerative colitis. The two illnesses are closely related, with similar, sometimes identical symptoms, but Crohn's is the more serious and is more likely to be the forerunner of bowel cancer. Since the term IBD does not discriminate between the illnesses, the older name, Crohn's disease, is generally used.

WHY DOES CROHN'S DISEASE MATTER SO MUCH?

- From Dr. Crohn's time onward, the illness has become increasingly prevalent, with occurrences doubling between 1930 and 1970 and more than tripling since then.

- The key symptoms of pain and diarrhea are unpleasant and socially embarrassing at best, exhausting, often disabling, and sometimes life-threatening at worst.

- New cases are appearing every day in increasing numbers, and these tend to become chronic, with ups and downs over the years.

- The most susceptible group is between ten and 40 years old, with a peak in the mid-twenties—years that are normally the most active and productive of one's life and among the happiest.

- While only three or four years ago the onset of Crohn's in people under age ten or over age sixty was almost unknown, now such occurrences are more and more common.

- Crohn's tends to affect people in countries with a Western culture, but we do not know exactly where the risk lies to enable us to avoid it. We know it is unrelated to social class or poverty. The one odd clue is that it is more likely to develop in people who were well fed—not overfed—as babies. A theory put forward in 1999 blaming the water supplies is not generally accepted.

• It can cause lasting damage to the developmental process if it occurs in children. Youngsters with untreated Crohn's disease are liable to be short and sexually immature.

• There is no quick-fix cure, despite a range of positive options for treatment.

• Getting the best out of life when you have this illness means reengineering your whole lifestyle.

HOW THIS BOOK CAN HELP

The maxim applies to many illnesses, but to Crohn's especially: the sooner the problem is recognized and treatment begun, the better the results, long-term and short. In conjunction with expert medical care from a team of health-care providers whom the patient trusts and has a rapport with, this book can help the reader to recognize and select among the strategies available for living with Crohn's. A doctor can offer advice, but ultimately any treatment decision is up to the patient. Being as well informed as possible is therefore essential. *Positive Options for Crohn's Disease* can help the reader—whether a Crohn's patient or a patient's family member or friend—know what questions to ask and thus make better treatment decisions.

The first few chapters discuss the disease's origins and its symptoms. Chapter 1 begins with a description of how the digestive process works under normal conditions and how the process is interrupted by Crohn's. Chapters 2 and 3 discuss the risk factors (including some statistics) and the signs and symptoms associated with Crohn's. These can help the reader in asking the right questions to assist the physician in making a proper diagnosis. Crohn's disease affects people of different ages in different ways, with special impact on seniors and youth. Chapters 4 and 5 describe the effects of the disorder on these two age groups. Because a well-functioning digestive system is such an important aspect of good health, when it fails to work properly it leaves the body unable to nourish itself optimally. If that happens, symptoms outside the digestive system can show up, for instance skin disorders, arthritis, or anemia. These possible effects of Crohn's are covered in chapter 6.

Finally we come to what the patient can expect in the doctor's office and in the hospital. Chapter 7 begins with a description of the tests that might be used to make a diagnosis. Chapters 8 through 10 describe the treatment options—utilizing both medicines and surgery—and their aftereffects, paying special attention to the two most "notorious" operations: ileostomy and colostomy. By offering straightforward, detailed, practical advice about life after these procedures, and by featuring real-life stories of ostomy patients (who have undergone one of these two procedures) who thrive—and improve—after these surgeries, the book can help alleviate the anxiety of any reader who may be facing such a procedure.

Diet is addressed in chapters 11 through 13, describing a healthful diet for the prevention of Crohn's, as well as giving detailed descriptions of typical dietary treatments of the disorder. This includes a discussion of the elemental diet, which provides all the essential nutrition through a liquid that contains no food at all, but is made of the nutritious components of food. This section concludes with pointers to help the reader—under the guidance of a physician or dietician—construct a personalized eating plan.

It is increasingly difficult to draw a hard and fast line between physical illness and its psychological causes and effects. Living with a chronic disorder usually affects one's mind and spirit. Chapter 14 discusses the mental and emotional aspects of Crohn's, including several options for dealing with depression or anxiety. Finally, chapter 15 covers the research occurring today to determine with certainty what causes Crohn's—research whose ultimate goal is to find a cure for this chronic disorder.

A special feature of *Positive Options for Crohn's Disease* is its many true case studies. These tell the inspiring stories of real people who, by working with their health-care teams to select the treatment options that work best for them, have learned to manage their Crohn's so that they can continue leading productive, fulfilling lives. One or more of these stories may especially resonate with you, offering a point of view or an idea that you may find useful or inspiring.

Together in this book we will explore what you can do to get the very best out of life with Crohn's: the healthiest lifestyle to lead and the various tricks and strategies you can use to beat this modern illness.

Chapter 1

The Digestive System: How It Works

I magine a life without eating and drinking—it wouldn't be much fun at all. You would miss out on a recurrent pleasure, a comfort in distress, and the focus of much of our social life, from a formal banquet or a candlelit supper for two to pizza with the family. Yet, for happy eating, you need a digestive system in good working order. It has to perform the everyday chemical magic of turning pizza and apple pie, or whatever you choose, into blood, brain, and bone—all manufactured to your own individual specifications.

To accomplish this miracle, the different parts of the digestive system must coordinate their separate tasks. The timing is crucial: the food must pass down the alimentary tract (the pathway through the digestive system) at exactly the right rate for the processing of each of the varied ingredients of your meal—proteins, carbohydrates, and fats—to be completed. All of this would be pointless without the next stage, the absorption of the processed nutrients into the bloodstream, so that your body can use them. The main area for absorption is the small intestine, the part most seriously affected by Crohn's. The final task of the digestive system is the disposal of the waste matter—down the toilet.

Crohn's disease upsets all of this—absorption in particular, but also the basic work of digestion and elimination—including the time frame. To understand Crohn's it helps to know the main parts of the digestive system and what they do. Besides, it is a fascinating story.

THE ALIMENTARY TRACT

The system operates under computer control. The computer is your brain, and it keeps in touch with every part through the nervous system. The two ends of the alimentary tract, the mouth and the anus, work in response to your conscious decisions—to eat and to go to the toilet. All the rest comes under the influence of the autonomic (automatic) nervous system, and most of the activity is reflex, like a knee jerk. That is, given a particular stimulus, in this case tapping the front of your knee, your knee jerks automatically. You don't have to give it a thought.

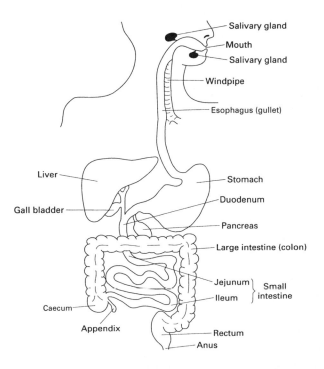

The alimentary tract: the pathway through the digestive system

Similarly, but in a much more complex way, the arrival of a steak or a piece of chicken in your stomach stimulates a reflex reaction in the stomach glands. They produce just the right amount of the digestive enzyme pepsin to digest the type and amount of protein. Imagine how tiresome it would be if you had to weigh and analyze what you ate, and then had to sit down with pencil and paper to work out which digestive enzymes you would need and the quantities. Instead, the whole system runs on a series of reflexes.

Although Burrill Crohn in the 1930s believed Crohn's could affect only the last few inches of the ileum, the terminal part, by the 1960s other doctors had found that the telltale patches of inflammation could show up anywhere in the alimentary tract. The effects—including your symptoms—differ according to the site of the trouble.

The Mouth

This is the entry point for food, where tasting and savoring help you to decide whether to go ahead and enjoy or spit it out. One job of the mouth is to smash and crunch up the food: this allows the digestive juices to reach all parts of it and also makes it easier to swallow. The other important task depends on the salivary glands, the saliva factories, which output about a quart per day. This slippery fluid lubricates each mouthful, making for easy transit down the esophagus (gullet) to the stomach. Saliva also contributes to oral hygiene by preventing crumbs of food sticking to the lining of the mouth and by washing away the germs that abound in the mouth.

Saliva has another useful role. It contains *ptyalin*, an enzyme that digests starch. You can test this out for yourself by chewing a piece of bread extra thoroughly. You will find it begins to taste sweet as the starch is digested into sugar. Our grandparents had a point when they advised us to chew every mouthful 32 times, making a mush with the saliva well mixed in and giving it time to work on the starch. An excellent start to digestion.

The salivary glands go into production when they receive information from the brain about the imminent arrival of food. My cat Emma dribbles in anticipation when she sees me open a can of cat food. Our human reflexes are similar, and we speak of something delicious as "mouth-watering." The actual presence of food in the mouth also promotes the flow of saliva. Another stimulus to the flow of saliva is when the stomach has been irritated and you feel nauseous. The extra saliva helps to flush out the harmful material, or at least dilutes it.

The Esophagus

This flexible, collapsible tube connects the mouth with the stomach. It is lined, like the whole of the alimentary tract, by moist, delicate mucous membrane. Mucous glands down its length provide it with a protective covering. Food does not just fall down from the mouth to the stomach, but is massaged along by the muscles in the wall of the esophagus. This is called *peristalsis* and is a feature of the whole alimentary tract. It makes it possible for circus performers to drink a glass of water while standing on their heads. You can feel the peristalsis working if you accidentally swallow a cherry pit or swallow a mouthful of food without chewing it.

The "law of the gut" is that throughout the alimentary tract, and most obviously in the esophagus and the intestines, peristalsis moves the contents continuously onward in the direction of the anus.

Lorna

Lorna had coped with her typical Crohn's quite effectively with the help of the standard drugs since age 22. It was when she was 28 that some new symptoms appeared. Swallowing became uncomfortable, then increasingly difficult, and she had an irritating cough. She lost about ten pounds and looked ill. X-rays and passing an endoscope into her esophagus showed Crohn's disease esophagitis, with numerous small ulcers and a narrowing caused by a ring of swollen, inflamed tissue mixed with scarring. The treatment consisted of gently stretching this area by passing bougies (pencil-shaped instruments for pushing into narrow or blocked tubes) of increasing size through it. After five sessions Lorna was able to swallow normally again. Her medication was also adjusted, and she soon entered a long period of remission.

The Stomach

As food travels down the esophagus a message flashes forward to the stomach: "Food on the way." The stomach muscles relax, especially at the entrance, and stomach glands begin to produce the appropriate digestive juices to deal with the type of food that is arriving.

The stomach serves several important functions:

1. As a storage chamber for large quantities of food, so that you do not have to chomp all the time like a cow, but can take in all you need for 24 hours at three or four meals.

2. Production of digestive juices, including hydrochloric acid to soften tough material, and *pepsin* to digest protein. This combination could be damaging to the body's own tissues, which is why there is a ring of muscle, the *pylorus*, that prevents the stomach contents from running back into the esophagus. The stomach lining is especially well coated with extrastrength mucous to protect it against the acid and pepsin. In the duodenum, just past the exit from the stomach, the bile duct pours out its secretions. Bile is strongly alkaline and neutralizes stomach acid. The stomach enzymes can digest carbohydrates as well as proteins.

3. Production of *intrinsic factor*, another constituent of the stomach juices. This is necessary for the absorption of vitamin B12, without which a serious form of anemia develops called pernicious anemia.

4. Kneading and thoroughly mixing the food and the stomach juices, for as long as necessary, to produce a milky-looking semifluid called *chyme*.

5. Slow, controlled emptying of the chyme into the small intestine, as and when facilities for the next stage become

available. There must obviously be room, and the rate of emptying is geared to allow for the digestive process to continue until the chyme is ready for absorption.

6. The correct rate of transit is of key importance to the digestive process, and nervous messages are sent both ways between the stomach and the small intestine to communicate, for instance, information that the chyme is still too acidic or contains too much undigested fat or protein—or is irritating for some other reason.

7. Stomach reflexes: the automatic message from the stomach to the small intestine is called the *gastroenteric reflex*, while the reverse, the *enterogastric reflex*, tells the stomach to turn off the production of acid and pepsin, because the chyme has moved into the intestine. (Any strong emotion has an equally powerful switch-off effect on the stomach.) Messages from the stomach to the colon set off the *gastrocolic reflex*. This alerts the colon to the arrival into the system of another meal, and this is often a good time to get rid of accumulated waste matter as, for instance, the after-breakfast bowel movement.

The Small Intestine

The small intestine comprises, in order, the duodenum, the jejunum, and the ileum. Its smallness refers to the relative narrowness of the tube compared with the much wider colon or large intestine, but it is many times longer. The gastroenteric reflex stimulates increased peristalsis in the small intestine, especially the jejunum. The normal travel time from the stomach through the small intestine to the caecum, where the large intestine begins, is between three and five hours, depending on the type and quantity of food in the system.

The *duodenum* is only a few inches long, little more than a lobby to the stomach. Partly because it is more exposed to the stomach juices than the lower parts of the intestine, ulcers often develop here. The most important role of the duodenum is the reception, through the bile duct, of digestive juices from the pancreas, and of bile made by the liver and stored in the gall bladder. The pancreatic enzymes aid in the digestion of all three kinds of foodstuff—proteins, fats, and carbohydrates. Bile is essential for the digestion and preparation for absorption of fats, a necessary requirement for the body to obtain its supplies of the fat-soluble vitamins: A, D, E, and K. The gall bladder automatically pours out all the bile it is storing when a fatty meal arrives in the duodenum.

The *jejunum* and *ileum* comprise the rest of the small intestine, coils many feet long. In the jejunum, located just after the duodenum, peristalsis is vigorous, and so are other muscular movements, ensuring that the chyme is thoroughly mixed with the digestive juices to make a runny mishmash. The digestive process continues as the chyme travels through the jejunum and is virtually complete when it reaches the ileum, the organ most affected by Crohn's. The ileum has the important task of absorbing almost all the nutrients from the chyme into the bloodstream, a role for which it is specifically adapted.

Its lining is covered with tiny, delicate fingers of tissue that both release liquid and reabsorb it when it is loaded with nourishment from the chyme. Another special feature of the cells lining the small intestine is their short life—five to seven days. The advantage of this is that any damage is quickly repaired with brand new cells, indicating how indispensable the ileum is to life. If there is some irritation in the small intestine, such as inflammation or the presence of bacteria, the movement of the chyme is speeded up, resulting in copious, watery diarrhea. This washes out germs or other irritants, but also causes the loss of essential nourishment.

Every day, when you are in normal health, your ileum absorbs into the bloodstream:

- several hundred grams of carbohydrate (100 g is equivalent to 3.5 ounces, or nearly a quarter pound)

- 100 g of fat

- 50–100 g of protein constituents (amino acids)

- 50–100 g of chemical ions, such as iron, calcium, and magnesium

- all the vitamins (naturally occurring compounds needed in small quantities for normal metabolism and bodily function, but which the human body cannot make for itself)

- 7–8 liters of fluid (a liter is the equivalent of about a quart)

The ileum is capable of absorbing much larger quantities if necessary: up to 20 liters of water in a day, for instance. Although the ileum is the main area for absorption, other parts of the digestive system can take in some substances. The stomach, for example, can absorb alcohol—the reason for its rapid effect—and several drugs, such as aspirin, and the duodenum absorbs calcium, so long as there is also some vitamin D available. The colon can only absorb water and a few simple chemicals dissolved in it.

The Large Intestine

The ileum ends in the *ileocaecal junction*, where there is a double ring of muscles to regulate when and at what rate the now depleted chyme is allowed through. It is reduced to about 1½ liters (1,500 ml) daily. The caecum is a bulge that marks the beginning of the large intestine. It is in the lower right-hand corner of the abdomen, and the appendix is a short dead-end alley that comes off it. The caecum continues as the colon until it becomes the specialized end section, the rectum, and the final exit, the anus.

The first half of the colon is called the "absorbing colon" since it absorbs most of the water and chemicals entering it, leaving about 100 ml for the waste mixture, the stool or feces. The second part is the "storage colon" where the waste is kept until there is a signal that it is time to empty it. There are normally many bacteria in the colon, especially "colon bacilli," and they are responsible for the gas or flatus that can be so embarrassing, produced from various foods such as beans, cabbage, and unabsorbable roughage.

The only material produced in the colon is mucous, and its lining is massed with mucous cells. These are stimulated by the presence of waste matter, and the mucous protects and lubricates the lining. It also helps to bind the waste—or fecal—matter together, for convenience in storage and disposal. The contents of the colon are semiliquid at the caecal end, mushy in the middle, and semisolid when they reach the rectum.

When the colon is irritated by inflammation, enteritis (inflammation of the ileum), or inadequately digested material, it reacts by pouring out more mucous and speeding up the passage of its contents by mass movements involving its whole length. Emotional disturbances stimulate the colon to produce a large amount of stringy mucous, which produces the urge to pass stool as often as every half hour—even if there is nothing to pass.

Andrew

Andrew was a conscientious 18-year-old, predictably nervous about final exams. He had always had a tendency to suffer from diarrhea when he was upset as a child, so no one took much notice when it happened this time. However, after one sharp attack the symptoms kept recurring, and he noticed that his stool contained bloodstained mucous and pus. Andrew had Crohn's disease affecting his colon, or Crohn's colitis. It responded well to a drug called sulfasalazine, an old favorite in the treatment of Crohn's.

The *rectum* and *anus* comprise the final parts of the alimentary tract and differ from the previous sections in that you have some conscious control over them. The sensitive rectum informs you when it is full and reminds you to go to the toilet. The muscle of the anus has to relax to allow the bowel movement to pass, and this is under your control so that you can wait for a convenient time and place. The anal region is especially sensitive, and inflammation here, *proctitis*, can be so painful that the sufferer may be afraid to let the stool pass.

The Bowel Movement

A normal stool consists of 75 percent water and 25 percent solids;

these in turn include 30 percent dead bacteria and their products, 30 percent indigestible fiber, and 10 to 20 percent fat. Too much water means diarrhea and too little leads to constipation, while an excess of fat gives a bulky, pale, putty-colored stool. Blood, pus, or mucous in the stool are all abnormal.

THE EMOTIONAL INPUT

No one would suggest that Crohn's and its serious symptoms are "all in the mind," but it would be unrealistic to claim that your feelings have no part to play in the working of your digestive system. It stands to reason that you cannot feel happy when you have stomach pain or diarrhea, but it is also true that emotional stress can bring on physical symptoms or make them worse.

Long before Sigmund Freud blamed bowel disorders on emotional conflict, or psychosomatic illnesses became fashionable in the 1950s, it was taken for granted that there was an intimate link between feelings and the bowels. In the Bible, Solomon, referring to a friend, said, "My bowels were moved for him," and St. John wrote of "the bowels of compassion." In the seventeenth century John Gay's MacHeath appealed to Lucy, "Have you no bowels, no tenderness?" while today, more crudely, we connect the bowels with courage. If we say that someone "hasn't got the guts for it," we are talking not anatomy but feelings.

Physicians and surgeons both focus on the physical aspects of Crohn's disease and argue over the relative merits of medicine and surgery in this illness. You, the sufferer, are in no position to join the argument on scientific grounds. Where you do have the edge is in the vast area of mind and emotions. Only you know your feelings, your hopes, your fears, and what you find stressful in your life. They cannot be analyzed chemically, X-rayed, or measured in milliliters, yet this part of you is involved in everything that happens in your body. The connection is obvious when you think of what happens when you are frightened or anxious. Your heart speeds up, your saliva dries up, and sometimes your bowels "turn to water."

You cannot switch on a calm, confident mood when you are feeling distressed, any more than you can will away a pain in your stomach or a bout of diarrhea. The psychological and emotional aspects of Crohn's require consideration as well as the physical side. Never forget that you are a whole person.

Chapter 2

Are You at Risk? The Background to Crohn's Disease

What are the risk factors for Crohn's disease, and is there anything you can do to lessen them? Unfortunately, it is not as simple with Crohn's as it is, for instance, with measles. In that case we know what causes it—the measles virus—and can alert our immunity system, or our children's, by vaccination. We have not pinpointed the cause of Crohn's, but we are fairly sure that it is a mix of several factors—none of which we know for certain. There are a few pointers, but no definite answers, despite the best endeavors of research workers over the last 70 years.

Epidemiology—the numbers game—can tell us how many people in different places and different circumstances develop the disease. This body count, since it affects whole communities, not just individuals, provides some clues about risk. It highlights the influence of race and family—the genetic input—compared with environmental factors such as lifestyle, stress, and diet.

The recent huge increase in the number of Crohn's cases in the West must be related to lifestyle rather than genetics—you cannot change your parents or your ancestry, but you can certainly change how and where you live. Your job, or your partner's, can take you to New York or New Delhi, or you may choose to move from town to country or vice versa—or become a vegetarian.

There must be something (or probably several things) in our so-called civilized Western way of life that makes us more susceptible to Crohn's than, for example, Zimbabweans or Nicaraguans. Whatever it is, it is getting worse. The importance of lifestyle on a countrywide basis is borne out by the increasing prevalence of Crohn's in the Western world and its even more dramatic upsurge in developing countries that are currently Westernizing, with industry replacing agriculture and a shift of population to the towns. This has been well documented in New Zealand, South Africa, and in the black population of the United States.

TOWN OR COUNTRY

All over Europe and the United States, where statistics have been collected, proportionately more cases of Crohn's are found in the towns, especially where there is much industry, than in rural areas. The instinct to retire to the country is a healthy one, but it comes too late to lessen the risk of Crohn's, since the peak age for developing it is 26.

DIET

No one type of diet, whether Mediterranean, Indian, vegetarian, plain American, or sophisticated French, is particularly associated with a higher or lower incidence of Crohn's disease. But there are a few significant dietary pointers.

Sugar

It has been shown recently in some countries that people with Crohn's disease habitually eat much more sugar than the average—150 percent more in Birmingham, England, 120 percent more in Tel Aviv, Israel, 110 percent more in Dusseldorf, Germany, and 40 percent more in Manchester, England. It is not certain whether the excess sugar makes Crohn's more likely or if the disease itself gives you a sweet tooth.

Fruits and Vegetables

Statistically, Crohn's disease sufferers eat far fewer servings of fruits and vegetables than other people. Twenty-five percent consume one portion or less of these foods daily, and hardly any meet the USDA-recommended guideline of five portions or more per day. (The USDA, short for United States Department of Agriculture, is the federal agency that sets dietary guidelines, among its other responsibilities.) This dietary deficiency is likely to have been a long-term pattern, present before the onset of Crohn's as well as after.

Fillers

Because of their low intake of green and yellow vegetables and of fruit, those who develop Crohn's are often heavy users of high-starch "filler" foods. They eat more potatoes, pasta, bread, cookies, cake, and breakfast cereals than the rest of us. At one time cornflakes came under the spotlight, but since they are usually eaten with milk and sugar, both also suspect, it was impossible to come to a firm conclusion about whether they were truly a risk factor.

Sometimes an entire extended family may go for the same old favorites: potatoes, cereal, chips, and cookies—with most things well sugared. Such families are more likely than others to include members who suffer from Crohn's and ulcerative colitis.

Processed Foods

Crohn's disease patients tend to go for convenience foods more than most. Can there, after all, be anything harmful in additives, preservatives, and flavor enhancers? Some people have a vague idea that with Crohn's the body is reacting to some mysterious, unidentified ingredient in our food—perhaps related to processing.

Poultry

Oddly, the only meats that seem relevant to the incidence of Crohn's are the ubiquitous chicken and turkey. These have

. become increasingly popular since red meat has experienced such bad press, and Crohn's patients eat more poultry than average. Much of it is bought in supermarkets, processed and packaged.

Dairy Products

Groups of researchers over the years have suspected dairy products as one of the roots of the trouble. In a study of American veterans with Crohn's, there were many more who stayed in remission (not permanently cured, but without symptoms) among a group who were not allowed dairy products, compared with those on full service rations. In the last five years there has been a serious suggestion that milk contaminated with Mycobacterium paratuberculosis is a prime cause of Crohn's. There is also the matter of lactase deficiency, a condition that seems to be pronounced in Crohn's sufferers and involves a shortage of the enzyme that breaks down milk sugar (see page 122). However, for many patients, disappointingly, cutting out this valuable nourishment seems to make no difference.

Caffeine

The habit of using an excess of this universal stimulant in coffee, tea, and cola drinks also slightly increases the risk of Crohn's disease.

Food Intolerance

Intolerance of certain foods may underlie Crohn's in some cases (see page 121). The evidence is indirect and comprises miraculous improvement for some people if a particular item of food is removed from their diet. It is not that Crohn's is an allergic reaction, since quite large quantities of food are required to bring on the symptoms. In fact a trial lasting seven days is now standard for testing for food intolerance. The food being tested is disguised in a fruit drink or a soup—or even delivered straight into the stomach through a tube—so there is no preconceived bias. A positive reaction is the appearance of Crohn's symptoms: pain and diarrhea. A wide range of foods has been implicated. The list below gives percentages of Crohn's patients who reacted positively in a food test.

wheat	28%
dairy products	24%
brassicas, cabbage family	16%
maize, corn	12%
yeast	11%
tomatoes	11%
citrus fruits	10%
eggs	10%
tap water, coffee, bananas, potatoes, lamb	8%
pork	7%
beef, rice	5%
tea	4%
fish	3%
onions	2%
chicken, barley, rye, turkey, alcohol, chocolate, shellfish, rutabaga, additives	1%

The patient is put on an elemental diet (see page 124), and different foods are reintroduced one by one, stopping the process if there is pain or diarrhea. In two-thirds of the cases, patients who respond favorably to diet changes are still well two years later.

Some theorize that it is not the particular food itself that sets off Crohn's disease, but rather its effect on the bacteria that normally inhabit the gut.

Philip

Philip was short for his twelve years when he developed Crohn's disease. His mother had a full-time job, and he was an only child. He was an independent youngster and took pride in managing for himself when his mother was at work. He could have chosen a snack of bread and cheese and helped himself from the fruit dish when he was hungry, but what he went for were chips, chocolate bars, and sometimes a bowl of sugar-frosted cornflakes. Even on weekends, when his mother cooked meals of a meat and two vegetables, Philip preferred ham from a packet, with chips, followed by a gooey sweet. His choice of food did nothing to hinder the development of Crohn's. However, diet alone could not have been responsible for the illness: there must also have been other genetic or environmental factors at work.

SMOKING

It has been found that the proportion of smokers among Crohn's sufferers is higher than average. This applies to their current smoking habit and also to what it was before the illness came on. The link with tobacco is stronger in the towns and cities of the U.K. than, for instance, in Chicago or Denver. The risk is cumulative, so the more heavily a person smokes or the longer he or she has been a smoker, the greater the risk. For an average smoker (1–2 packs a day) the risk increases four times, not only the risk of developing the disease in the first place but also the chances of recurrence, and it is likely to be more serious. Furthermore, the likelihood of needing surgery (see chapters 9 and 10 for details of surgical options) is greater for Crohn's patients who continue smoking.

THE CONTRACEPTIVE PILL

Women on oral contraceptives sustain an increased risk of Crohn's disease, particularly if they are taking a high-estrogen formula. Back in 1968, when the pill was still under close scrutiny, it was discovered that, like smoking, the pill was associated in some mysterious way with damage to the tiny blood vessels in the lining of the colon. There was an increased risk of Crohn's, especially of the colon rather than the ileum.

In one study, 75 percent of women age 40 or younger who had Crohn's were on the pill, compared with 31 percent of other women in the same age range. The risk of Crohn's is doubled for those on the pill, and if they have taken it for more than five years the risk is up to eight times the norm. On the other hand, if they stop taking it the extra risk declines to nothing over five years.

HRT (HORMONE REPLACEMENT THERAPY)

Since this treatment for postmenopausal women contains the same hormones as the oral contraceptive pill, it seems likely that it carries the same risks, but there are fewer cases of Crohn's disease in the middle-aged than in the young, so people in this age group figure less in research studies.

CONSTIPATION

Long-term constipation, with the nonstop use of laxatives, is considered by some to predispose the patient to both IBD and irritable bowel syndrome. However, constipation is so widespread among normal, healthy people that its effect on the incidence of Crohn's would be negligible.

Kirsty

Kirsty liked to live life to the fullest. She had begun smoking at 13 and drinking alcohol at about the same time, and she went on the pill almost as soon as her period started. By age 35, twice divorced and with a successful career as a secretary-turned-administrator under her belt, she lost her appetite and dropped seven pounds without trying. She felt tired—unusual for her—and her doctor, who knew Kirsty had a cousin with ulcerative colitis, referred her to a specialist. The specialist diagnosed IBD but did not subject her to unpleasant invasive investigations to see whether it was Crohn's or ulcerative colitis, since if her symptoms settled down there would be no definitive sign of either illness anyway.

Kirsty underwent several months of treatment with a battery of drugs. She stopped taking the pill and stopped smoking and with her positive spirit, rebuilt her life. She also remarried and began thinking of having children.

MICROORGANISMS (GERMS)

In 1913, Dr. Kennedy Dalziel identified an as yet unnamed illness in cows similar to Crohn's disease and caused by a mycobacterium very like, but not the same as, that which causes tuberculosis of the intestines in humans.

Seventeen years later, Dr. Crohn and his colleagues continued the hunt for a mycobacterium in the tissues of their Crohn's disease patients. Like a relay race, others took up the challenge, and in 1978 they struck oil. A group of four researchers found Mycobacterium paratuberculosis in the tissues of one patient with Crohn's (*para* means *like*, as in paramedic). In 1984, the microbe was found in four more patients, then in some macaque monkeys. The research took so many years because of the inordinate length of time—up to eight months—required for the mycobacterium to grow in the laboratory. Earlier workers must often have given up hope of any bacteria developing. Now we have the recipe for a culture medium that this persnickety bug really likes: veal broth with yeast extract, horse serum, sugar, and a few other choice ingredients.

Mycobacterium paratuberculosis and one of its close relatives are found in as many as a third of Crohn's patients. This must mean that it is implicated in some way. Further evidence of mycobacterial involvement is the occasional dramatic improvement in the patient's symptoms using antimycobacterial antibiotics such as streptomycin, and in the last two years lesser-known drugs such as rifabutin. The big problem is the lack of consistency in study results. Viruses have also been investigated for a link to Crohn's, and some unusual organisms, such as Pseudomonas, have come under suspicion, but studies have been disappointingly inconclusive.

Another germ theory is that Crohn's patients have a fault in the lining of the gut, which allows bacteria that normally cause no trouble to penetrate the surface and produce the patches of inflammation that comprise the disease. Suspect bugs include Streptococcus faecalis and E. (Escherichia) coli and, of course, Mycobacterium paratuberculosis. The weakness of the lining membrane would be a genetic condition present from birth.

Rather than any particular microorganism causing Crohn's directly, it is more likely that certain ones predispose the person to the illness and only trigger it when there are other influences at work—faults in the gut lining or in the immune system, or some of the adverse dietary and lifestyle factors. A large number of people may, for instance, be harboring the mycobacterium, but only a few develop the symptoms. Some people may be hypersensitive to the particular microbe, or their immune system has in some way been primed to react in the wrong way.

A natural phenomenon that can confuse the issue is that different causes may produce the same effect on the body. For example, we all know that a headache may be the result of alcohol or another drug, a migraine, a sinus infection, a stuffy room, or anxiety. In Crohn's there may need to be more than one adverse factor acting together to produce the disorder.

DEFECTS IN THE IMMUNE SYSTEM

Another current notion proposes that Crohn's disease is an abnormal reaction by the immune system, either to something that is normally harmless, or perhaps to a toxin left behind by a germ that has passed through the body. All this is speculative, but a great deal of work is in progress, and researchers are keeping their fingers crossed.

STEROID MEDICINES

To add to the confusion, while steroid medicines often suppress Crohn's disease symptoms in the short term, if they are used continuously their long-term effects actually reduce the chances of remission. (This is in contrast to the wholly beneficial effect of steroids in ulcerative colitis, the other IBD.)

GENETICS

Important as environmental factors are, genes have an enormous individual effect. If you have a brother or sister with Crohn's, you run 30 times the risk of developing the illness compared with the general population—and a staggering 67 times if you are identical twins. The risk is only about 13 times greater if you have a parent or other first-degree relative with the illness; this applies equally to your offspring. One curious fact is that if you suffer from Crohn's you are more likely to have relatives with ulcerative colitis than with Crohn's itself.

These risks may sound alarming, but to get them in perspective remember that the chances of developing Crohn's for the general population are small—about 16 out of 100,000 people per year. Even multiplied by 30, this does not amount to many. Of course there are more Crohn's cases in the most vulnerable age group, those in their mid-twenties, but even among these the numbers are relatively small. In 1996 among all those aged 26 in the U.K., the proportion diagnosed as having Crohn's came out at 30 per 10,000.

Sex, which is a genetic factor, makes no difference to your likelihood of getting Crohn's, apart from one small, fairly rare group where sex is indirectly involved. In these cases the gene passes from mother to son only, the so-called X-linked inheritance. For these Crohn's sufferers the illness always starts up in childhood and often affects a large part of the small intestine.

A more dramatic genetic link affects the whole Jewish population, particularly the Ashkenazi line (those of European descent). American Ashkenazi Jews are four to five times more likely to develop IBD than the general population; the rates among Jews in other countries are even higher, between eight and thirteen times the normal risk. This seems to be based on a metabolic quirk, also genetic. They tend to have a shortage of lactase, an enzyme used in the digestion of milk. Although this suggests that milk products should be avoided, by Jewish people especially, it is only one factor among many and may have an insignificant effect by itself. Of the Western countries, Israel has the greatest proportion of Crohn's sufferers, partly due to the genetic effect, but also because it is still actively developing industrially.

Rachel

Rachel's grandparents had left Germany just in time in 1939, and by a circuitous route reached Australia. Rachel was a third-generation Aussie, fit and athletic. She excelled at swimming and was a junior champion at one time. Naturally, she led a healthy lifestyle—no cigarettes, plenty of fruit and vegetables, moderate alcohol, and regular exercise—so it came as a shock when she developed Crohn's disease. There had been some question of an uncle of hers having a serious bowel problem, but he was in Europe and not in close touch. A distant cousin was prone to bouts of diarrhea, but she had been discounted as "neurotic." There was no doubt about the seriousness of Rachel's illness, however, and she required an urgent operation. Her excellent health stood her in good stead in this crisis, and she made a smooth recovery from her surgery, which successfully removed the affected part of her small intestine. She is now back in training—after several months of concentrating solely on her recovery.

PSYCHOLOGICAL AND EMOTIONAL RISK FACTORS

It cannot be doubted that there is interplay between psychological events and physical symptoms, but for Crohn's disease it is not a simple matter of cause and effect. Some personality types and some less permanent emotional states, such as depression or anxiety, may predispose one to Crohn's, and some stressful events may hasten an attack, particularly when one already has the illness.

Psychological shocks and strains may act as triggers, for example, losing a loved one, getting divorced, being robbed, accumulating debt, starting a new job, or losing a job. Physical stresses may also act as triggers, such as a severe infection, pregnancy, or starting menstrual periods. Even happy events, like getting married or winning the lottery, act as stressors, and for Crohn's sufferers the bowels are the weak spot.

People who develop Crohn's disease are usually stable, conscientious, and reliable; they are not given to exaggeration or complaining unnecessarily. In fact, although they are sensitive, they tend to hide their hurt. Like anyone else, if you fall into a depression or an anxiety state, you are more vulnerable to illness, and this includes Crohn's. Equally, it lowers one's spirits to suffer an attack of the disease and to live with anxiety about the outcome.

The psychological aspects of Crohn's are touched upon in chapters 1 and 10 and are dealt with more fully in chapter 14.

Leonard

Leonard was a teacher at a primary school. At 24 he had been teaching for only a year when the abdominal pains began. He tried to ignore them. He had always wanted to teach and to share the pleasure he derived from his chosen subject, history. He found his life at the school was a roller coaster of delights and disasters, with the emphasis on the latter. Despite the constant pain, he managed to cope with the day-to-day hurdles until he succumbed to a nasty bout of flu. While recovering from it the bowel symptoms came out in full force. The depression that commonly follows influenza merged with his depression over contracting Crohn's disease. His bowel symptoms and his depression both required treatment. A steroid for the former and an antidepressant for the latter enabled him to return to a productive life.

The causes of Crohn's are *multifactorial*—that is, there must be a concurrence of several different factors, genetic and environmental, acting together to enable the disease to develop. But the good news, as some of our case examples have already demonstrated, is that very often the symptoms can be managed successfully by finding and applying the appropriate combination of treatment options.

Chapter 3

Signs and Symptoms: How Crohn's Disease Manifests Itself

Crohn's disease, although not a killer, is troublesome enough to interfere with your life disastrously—if you let it. So the sooner the illness is diagnosed and treatment is started the better: you suffer less and learn to adapt to the lifestyle that suits you best. The first step is up to you. If you notice anything unusual or uncomfortable about your bowels or your abdomen that does not settle down in a few days, especially if you have any of the symptoms listed below, do not bravely ignore them. Have them checked out. It will probably turn out to be nothing of importance, but it is worthwhile to be sure.

Crohn's can appear in several different guises. Usually it comes on insidiously, creeping up almost imperceptibly and either getting gradually but steadily worse or manifesting in little bouts of symptoms that become increasingly frequent. Less often there is a sudden, explosive start to the illness, with dramatic symptoms of pain, vomiting, and diarrhea.

COMMON SYMPTOMS

The three most common symptoms are pain, diarrhea, and under-nutrition. These key symptoms may not be the first warning signs, however. Look out for any of the following:

Pain in the Abdomen

In Crohn's this is likely to be in the lower right-hand corner, the appendix area. Most frequently it is constant rather than throbbing or colicky. Often you can notice a slight fullness, not quite a bulge, in the area, and it may be tender to pressure. This is due to the pain and swelling of inflamed tissues, particularly the peritoneum, the sensitive membrane which covers the intestines.

If there is a degree of obstruction in the intestine, causing a build-up of its contents, the intestine wall is stretched, and this registers as pain. Slight, partial obstruction may be due to the inflamed lining itself, a band of tough, fibrous scar tissue, or muscle spasm. In the colon and rectum such spasms are called *colorectal cramps*. Muscle spasms can also occur in the small intestine or the esophagus. They may be set off by inflammation or by the irritation of incompletely digested food arriving in the affected part, but typically they are a symptom of the muscle pushing hard to get material past a narrow or more seriously blocked section of the gut. In this situation the pain is colicky and is felt in the center of the abdomen.

"Tummy Rumbles"

These may be loud and excessive if your intestinal muscles are having to work extra hard to keep things moving. Their scientific name is *borborygmi*.

Poor Appetite (Anorexia)

Everything may taste different or seem to have no taste or smell—or at any rate not an appetizing one—and you feel full after only a few mouthfuls. There is no pleasure in eating.

Nausea

If nausea develops you will not feel at all like eating. Anorexia, nausea, and sometimes diarrhea may all be caused by a lack of vitamins or trace minerals like zinc: a vicious circle if you are not eating properly. A more likely cause for nausea, however, is a direct effect of Crohn's on your stomach and duodenum. In 8 percent of people with Crohn's there are visible signs of the trouble if the doctor looks into the stomach with a flexible fiber-optic telescope: a process called endoscopy. In 24 percent there is an abnormal X-ray.

In Crohn's disease the stomach passes the food into the small intestine more slowly than normal. This is due to the "ileal brake." The ileum is almost always affected and cannot absorb the nourishment in your food effectively. This means that the material the ileum passes on is not fully digested and it irritates the colon at the ileocaecal junction. The ring of muscle there clamps down to slow, if not completely prevent, the flow of irritating stuff. This slowdown or "brake" produces a pressure all the way back to the stomach. The whole system of appetite, eating, and being nourished is upset, a measure of how important this illness is.

Vomiting

This may be a symptom of obstruction of the gut, or part of an acute phase, when the whole digestive system is in turmoil.

Lump in the Abdomen

Sometimes Crohn's patients—or their doctor—can feel a definite lump in the painful part of the abdomen. This is made up of coils of small intestine stuck together by the inflammatory process. It is not a cancer and is not serious in itself.

Elevated Temperature

A temperature increase goes with any inflammation, but is likely to be slight in Crohn's, unless it arises in the type that comes on acutely. The average normal temperature is between 98 and 98.6°F.

Malaise

This comprises a vague feeling of being unwell, or "having an off day"—which goes on and on. Even if there is nothing definitely wrong, you just do not feel right.

Diarrhea

Crohn's patients have frequent bowel movements. These may be loose and semiliquid or fully formed, bulky, and pale, but the daily quantity is well above normal. Diarrhea may originate in either the small or the large intestine. A large volume of liquid, passed with more inconvenience than pain, suggests that the ileum is to blame. If there is pain, with blood, pus, and mucous in the feces, the colon is directly involved. There may be an uncomfortable feeling in the rectum all the time, with a strong urge to pass a stool and only a little mucus to show for the effort (*tenesmus*).

Other Abdominal Symptoms

Crohn's sufferers may have any of these symptoms:

- Bloating, so that the abdomen seems enormous, except first thing in the morning.

- An excessive urge to pass gas.

- Dyspepsia—discomfort after meals.

- Heartburn.

Undernutrition

This means a lack of essential nourishment. It arises in Crohn's sufferers for three main reasons:

- Eating too little because of poor appetite.

- Losing nourishment through diarrhea and vomiting.

- Failure of the small intestine to absorb properly most of the major nutrients—carbohydrates, fats, and proteins—as well as the equally essential vitamins and minerals, even though only tiny amounts of these are necessary. If your ileum is ill and unable to work normally--the situation in Crohn's—it does not matter how well balanced your diet is, you cannot get the goodness from it.

Shortness of Stature

This is noticeable in those in whom the disease began to develop before or during their adolescent growth spurt. Sometimes the illness starts quietly long before the telltale symptoms appear.

Eileen

Eileen was a 20-year-old student who kept getting a pain in the right side of her abdomen. One day it was worse than usual and she felt generally lousy, so she took her temperature and found that it was slightly elevated at 99.7°F. She decided to consult the college doctor. He found Eileen's appendix area tender, and he also detected some guarding, a protective tightening of the muscles over the place that was hurting. Eileen felt sick but she did not vomit. The doctor sent her to the hospital with a provisional diagnosis of acute appendicitis.

At the hospital a blood test showed an excess of white cells (*leukocytosis*) such as occurs in appendicitis and other inflammatory conditions. The commonplace operation of appendectomy seemed the obvious thing to do. During the surgery the surgeon found that Eileen's appendix was perfectly healthy, but the last few inches of her ileum were swollen and sore. The inflammation was well established, healing in some parts while spreading in others, so it must have been developed over several months without Eileen's realizing anything was amiss. The surgeon took a tiny sample of the affected tissue, which confirmed what he had suspected—that Eileen had Crohn's disease. The operation did no harm and uncovered the real diagnosis. Treatment was started immediately, in this case with sulfasalazine, a well-tried standby in Crohn's.

Debbie

Debbie was in sales. She was 38 and had always been slim but recently had experienced several bouts of diarrhea and lost a few pounds. That was why she was so distressed to find her abdomen blowing up whenever she had a meal, so that it bulged out—"as though I was pregnant," she complained. Her doctor tried various things but they did not help, and he finally sent Debbie to a gastroenterologist. The specialist arranged a special type of X-ray involving a barium infusion (see page 65) which showed ulcers in the lining of the ileum and a narrowing (*stenosis*) in one section. These were the clues to the diagnosis of Crohn's disease.

The first medication Debbie was given was a steroid, which settled her abdomen quickly, and this was followed by azathioprine, a better treatment for the long term.

MALABSORPTION

The principal feature of Crohn's disease is damage to the small intestine so that it cannot do its job of absorbing the nourishment from food. This is malabsorption.

Effects of malabsorption

- Loss of weight in adults.

- Slowing of growth and development in children, particularly growth in height and sexual development.

- Loss of protein, which sets off a vicious circle of diarrhea and increased weight loss, with muscle weakness and wasting; there may also be swelling of the ankles and hands and sometimes the face.

- Passing of undigested fat in the stool, involving the loss of the important fat-soluble vitamins, A and D.

- Inadequate absorption of carbohydrates, the major filler in the diet, and the usual fuel for running the brain and all the body processes. Milk sugar, called lactose, is particularly poorly absorbed because of a deficiency in the necessary enzyme, lactase. Some Crohn's sufferers are intolerant to milk products and react to them with colic, bloating, gas, and sometimes diarrhea.

Vitamin and Mineral Deficiencies

Vitamin A (Retinol): A lack can cause dry, uncomfortable eyes and "night blindness"—poor vision in twilight conditions. Vitamin A has been called the anti-infection vitamin because it helps to protect the mucous membranes, for instance in the throat and the alimentary tract, from infection.

Vitamin D (Calciferol): A shortage produces an inability to absorb and use calcium, which is necessary for the health and strength of bones and teeth.

Vitamin B12 (Cobalamin): It is needed for the formation of red blood corpuscles. A lack leads to a serious form of anemia, called pernicious anemia, whose symptoms include weakness and tiredness, pale skin, sore tongue, and bouts of diarrhea. The nervous system, including the brain, may be affected.

Folate: This acts in conjunction with vitamin B12. A lack of either increases the effects of a lack of the other.

Iron: A deficiency leads to simple anemia, with such symptoms as fatigue, dizziness, shortness of breath, palpitations, headache, dim vision, and swollen ankles—but often these symptoms are slight and are ignored.

Magnesium: This is required by the nerves that service the muscles. A lack leads to a tremor and odd, involuntary muscular movements, and sometimes depression or a muddled feeling. It plays a key role in the metabolism of sugars and starches.

Calcium: A shortage in adults leads to osteoporosis, and in children to weak, faulty bones (rickets) and poor teeth.

Zinc: A deficiency can cause diarrhea, eczema around the mouth, and general apathy. In children growth and sexual development in particular are stunted.

For practical purposes, if you have any vague symptoms of tiredness or muscle weakness and you have been losing weight over a matter of weeks, it is worthwhile discussing with your doctor whether you should have a check for deficiency of any of these vitamins and minerals.

WHEN THE COLON IS AFFECTED

Often both the small intestine and the colon (large intestine) are involved in Crohn's disease, and in a minority the colon only is affected—Crohn's colitis. Crohn's colitis is almost indistinguishable from ulcerative colitis, the other IBD.

The symptoms are:

- Diarrhea (the key symptom), with blood, pus, and mucous in the stool. Blood is particularly likely in people over age 40. In the occasional case, there is constipation instead of diarrhea.

- Fast heart rate (*tachycardia*), felt in the chest and by counting the pulse. More than 90 beats a minute is abnormally fast unless you are exercising.

- High, fluctuating temperature, highest in the evening.

- Swollen, tender abdomen.

- Tenesmus—you feel you want to pass a stool even when there is nothing there.

- Edema—swelling due to waterlogging of the tissues, affecting your ankles and hands. If you press your finger into the swollen part, it leaves a little pit that takes a few seconds to go back to normal.

- Tags of swollen (*edematous*) skin around the anus.

Crohn's colitis usually comes on as an acute attack with the symptoms at their worst. It may be mistaken for food poisoning—gastroenteritis—initially, but in the case of Crohn's there is a tendency for the illness to persist and become chronic. The acute symptoms die down but do not disappear completely. Every now and then there is an acute exacerbation, but these recurrences are hardly ever as severe as the first attack.

Daniel

Daniel, 50, thought he "had eaten something" when he was suddenly seized with diarrhea streaked with blood and his whole abdomen felt sore and tender. His temperature was nearly 106.3°F. His doctor thought gastroenteritis was the likeliest cause but took a stool sample and reassured Daniel that he expected the symptoms to settle down within 48 to 72 hours. They did not, and the stool sample did not contain salmonella or any of the other common culprits. The doctor then referred Daniel to the nearest major hospital, where a colonoscopy (fiber-optic examination of the colon) was carried out. It showed the "cobblestone" appearance of the lining of the colon, characteristic of Crohn's disease. After an initial treatment of steroids, Daniel did well on loperamide.

COMMON MISDIAGNOSES

Sometimes Crohn's may at first "look like" other ailments, causing doctors to mistake it for another disease until further tests are performed. Some of these more common disorders are:

- Gastroenteritis or food poisoning, as in Daniel's case.

- Ulcerative colitis: sometimes only a biopsy can distinguish it from Crohn's. A biopsy entails taking a sample of the gut lining and examining it under the microscope.

- Acute appendicitis, as in Eileen's case.

- Peptic ulcer.

- Bowel cancer.

- Abdominal tuberculosis.

Fortunately, there are various tests and investigations, particularly special types of X-rays and endoscopy and sometimes ultrasound, to help doctors to make sure they have the right diagnosis (see chapter 7). Several conditions may crop up in the course of Crohn's with symptoms outside the digestive system. It is important to recognize these as related to the Crohn's process and deal with them accordingly. Examples are arthritis, including severe back problems, conjunctivitis and other eye disorders, and various skin troubles. These are dealt with in detail in chapter 6.

A FEW DEFINITIONS

The terms below appear frequently in the book, so a brief explanation is given here.

Fistula

A *fistula* (Latin for tube) is an abnormal and unwanted passage from one organ to another, formed by ulceration from an affected part breaking through to another organ—for instance from the colon to the bladder, vagina, or womb—or another section of gut.

Ileostomy and Colostomy

These are surgical procedures, discussed in more detail in chapter 10, which create an artificial opening in the front of the abdomen through which a person will need to pass their bowel movements because of an obstruction in the normal passage. The new exit is called a *stoma* (Greek for mouth). An ileostomy connects to the small intestine; a colostomy connects to the colon. In the case of a colostomy the stoma is usually made below and to the left of the navel, while an ileostomy stoma is placed low down on the right.

Skip Areas

These are patches of Crohn's disease, usually in the small intestine, with areas of normal tissue intervening.

Chapter 4

Children and Adolescents

The proportion of youngsters, even babies, developing Crohn's has been increasing ever since the disease was recognized. Nowadays about a third of cases are diagnosed before the age of 21, with 12 percent under age 15. Just as with adults, Crohn's is most prevalent among youngsters living in urban industrial settings.

Official statistics always lag behind events, but we know that in 1974 ten children in every 100,000 developed Crohn's each year in the U.K., and that this was four times as many as in 1959. Those living in the U.K. who are most at risk are Afro-Caribbean, Indian, and Jewish children.

A recent report shows that for the first time, the incidence of Crohn's disease in young people from urban Sweden appears to be on the rise. The rate of new cases in Stockholm County has nearly doubled in the last few years, rising from 2.9 per 100,000 in 1993–1995 to 5.4 per 100,000 in 1996–1998. Although new cases in children and youths have been increasing in other parts of the developed world, this is the first time any such increase has been reported in Scandinavia.

In the United States, 10 percent, or an estimated 100,000, of those afflicted with IBD of either type (Crohn's disease or ulcerative colitis) are under age 18.

The special, defining characteristic of childhood Crohn's is the disruption of growth and development, due almost entirely to lack of nourishment.

HOW THE ILLNESS MAY BE
RECOGNIZED IN CHILDREN

Failure to Grow at the Normal Rate

As in adults, Crohn's disease usually comes to notice because of abdominal pain, diarrhea, and undernutrition, the last being the most important. But while adults lose weight, children, instead, experience a slowing of their growth rate. This can easily go unnoticed for some time, or be dismissed with "he's a late developer," especially since the abdominal symptoms may not appear at first. Kind friends and even doctors are likely to reassure worried parents that their child "is growing at his or her own pace" and that puberty will eventually proceed normally and the lag in growth will correct itself. Partly because of this attitude, the diagnosis of Crohn's in children is delayed on average by three years from the onset of the first indications of the disorder. Growth in height is most severely affected and is the most obvious.

Once Crohn's disease has been suspected, the diagnosis can be confirmed by X-rays or endoscopy (see chapter 7).

Loss of Weight

If undernutrition and failure to grow properly are allowed to continue, a child may begin to lose weight. This is a serious symptom in a child who should be growing.

Failure to Develop Sexually

If Crohn's strikes before puberty, sexual development is delayed. This can be very embarrassing for a teenager at school, and more important, if the sex organs remain immature for too long, the boy or girl will have difficulty forming teenage relationships and may be unable to have children later.

Crohn's of the Mouth

Symptoms affecting the two ends of the digestive system, the mouth and the anus, occur more often in the young than in adults. Crohn's disease of the mouth is especially troublesome. There may be painful cracks, ulcers, and fissures in the mucous membrane lining the mouth and, most distressing of all, swelling, ulceration, and fissuring of the lips, the "thick lip syndrome." It seldom occurs in adults, while in children with Crohn's it is a frequent cause of a refusal to eat—adding to the other causes of undernutrition.

Unfortunately the steroid ointments that are so effective in most skin disorders do very little for "thick lip," but steroids by mouth can be helpful, if used with care (see page 46). In extreme cases, where it is urgent to get some nourishment into the child, tube feeding may be necessary (see chapter 11).

Jamie

Jamie was 11 when he began saying he had a "stomachache" and having bouts of diarrhea. He must have had "silent" Crohn's for some time, because in spite of having quite tall parents, he was short for his age and showed no signs of approaching puberty. He was one of the unlucky ones who developed Crohn's of the mouth, oral Crohn's disease, and for a short period—before beginning treatment—he could only take nourishment through a straw. Ointment was useless, but steroid medication by mouth helped both his oral and his abdominal symptoms to subside.

The snag for children is that steroid medicines, like Crohn's itself, hold back normal growth and cannot be used freely.

Jamie's Crohn's disease had come on at a time of family tension, when his parents were divorcing, but he slowly improved with treatment, when his home life with his mother became more settled. Both his parents were concerned about his sexually immature body, but when he managed to take in a generous diet, with supplements, his delayed puberty was normal when it arrived. At 18 Jamie is only a little shorter than average, and he has a very nice girlfriend.

Ano-rectal Crohn's

Symptoms affecting the anal passage, ano-rectal Crohn's, are sometimes the first manifestation of Crohn's disease in children and especially adolescents. They may precede the classic small-intestine disorder by several years. Perianal (around the anus) problems can be agonizingly embarrassing for those in the most sensitive period of their lives, teenagers. Leakage or discharge can be devastating to social activities and seriously inhibit the development of intimate relationships.

Saeed

Saeed, at 18, was his parents' pride and joy. After attending an inner-city high school he had obtained a place at a prestigious university and was all set for a sparkling career in science. This more than made up for his lack of prowess in sports, for Saeed was somewhat undersized and without much physical stamina. It was when it became excruciatingly painful to pass a bowel movement that he went reluctantly to the doctor.

The doctor did not like what he saw and started asking Saeed about his sexual orientation and experience, and if anyone had interfered with him sexually when he was younger. He also suggested an interview with Saeed's father. Saeed felt insulted. His sexual organs, like the rest of him, were undersized and his interest in that direction was lukewarm. What the doctor had seen were a few little pieces of skin hanging down around Saeed's anus, which he had thought at first were signs of sexual abuse—not an uncommon mistake in such cases. However, the doctor referred Saeed to the hospital, where the skin tags were recognized by a bright young resident as one of the characteristics of ano-rectal Crohn's. Microscopic examination of a biopsy sample from one of the tags confirmed the diagnosis. Saeed had no symptoms elsewhere in his body, but his poor physique and sexual immaturity indicated that the disease had been present for years, causing long-term undernutrition.

A steroid ointment and metronidazole controlled Saeed's problem moderately well, but he will probably opt for a surgical solution later.

Up to 95 percent of Crohn's sufferers find it preferable or necessary to undergo surgery sooner or later. The procedures and their objectives are described in chapters 9 and 10. When the diseased area has been removed, the child's—or adult's—quality of life takes a lasting upturn. Children are naturals for adapting to new situations, and they cope well, for instance, with an *ileostomy*, in which a loop of the ileum is brought to the surface and acts as an anus.

Diffuse Small-Intestine Crohn's Disease

Although the young are especially prone to developing Crohn's in the mouth or the anal passage, more show the usual adult symptoms of pain and diarrhea because of Crohn's of the intestines. Youngsters are unlucky in that nearly the whole of the ileum may be affected, a condition called *diffuse ileitis*, as opposed to the more common, patchy involvement. Diffuse small-intestine Crohn's is found in 13 percent of children with Crohn's, compared with 4 percent of adults with Crohn's, while proportionately fewer children have the illness confined to the colon.

The result is an even more serious degree of undernutrition—at a stage in life when more, rather than less, nourishment is required. The younger the child the more important this is.

FACTORS THAT STUNT GROWTH

- Inflammation or infection anywhere, especially accompanied by a raised temperature.

- Eating less because of anorexia, or to avoid pain in the mouth or from passing a bowel movement.

- Increased loss of nutrients from diarrhea, vomiting, bleeding, or the vicious-circle effect of protein loss, leading to greater inability to absorb it.

- Catch-up growth followed by a standstill.

- Lack of growth hormone.

- Side effects of certain medication, such as corticosteroids and sulfasalazine.

If parents do not check their child's height and weight regularly or accurately, they may miss the downward trend—or, more likely, the standstill—in growth caused by undernutrition.

TREATMENT IN CHILDREN AND YOUNG PEOPLE

The goals are:

- To suppress and then control the active disease.

- To get the child back on track with growth and development.

- To get enough nourishment into the child for all their needs, plus extra for catch-up growth and for puberty.

- To avoid or reduce, as far as possible, unpleasant symptoms or feelings, hospital admissions, time away from school.

- To minimize the side effects of medicines the child has to take.

- To avoid or reduce the use of steroids.

- To build up the child's self-confidence and encourage normal preteen and teenage clothes, appearance, interests, and activities with the peer group.

- To hold surgical treatment in reserve for acute situations.

Specific treatment includes various medicines, used particularly with a view to avoid having to take steroids more often than on alternate days, the elemental diet (see page 126), and other special diets with an emphasis on protein and calories in general, with supplements. Feeding may be administered by a tube into the stomach or by a vein when urgent building-up of nutrients is required.

Steroids (Corticosteroids)

These are the quickest and most effective medicines for halting the acute symptoms, but for children in particular they hold special dangers that must be weighed against the benefits. As little as 5 mg (milligrams) of prednisolone daily is enough to suppress normal growth. The bones are at special risk, and boys seem to be more susceptible than girls to a delay in the growing and maturing of the skeleton. There is a shortage of calcium (*osteopenia*) in the vertebrae that constitute the backbone. Long-term or continuous use of steroids must be avoided in children. See chapter 8 on drug treatments.

THE OUTLOOK FOR YOUR CHILD

Although they can be acutely ill for differing amounts of time, very few children die from Crohn's disease. What you can expect is a stormy period—illness-wise—around puberty, in addition to the normal early-teenage issues. Calmer waters follow. Although most children, like other Crohn's patients, will require surgery at some time in their lives, they do not have the same propensity that adults have for repeated severe attacks.

The absolutely vital element in managing Crohn's disease in a child is the attitude of the parents. The youngsters are bound to have emotional setbacks, frustrations, and disappointments at school and among their friends. They must learn to live with Crohn's and cope with the rough-and-tumble of life. They may find overconcerned, overprotective parents undermining. An anxiously hovering mom can do more harm than good by confirming how difficult life is with Crohn's, and how fraught with dangers. As a parent you must steel yourself not to show signs of worry, but to accept risk-taking and applaud all social activities that show the independence of the child.

The symptoms of Crohn's are, by their nature, infantilizing. You must do all you can to counteract this even if it means withholding help when you ache to give it, and not allowing too dependent a relationship to develop between you and your child. Independence is precious; it comes from having to manage for oneself at a level just past what seems possible. No other way stretches both capabilities and confidence.

Professional Help

Counseling or skilled psychotherapy can help your child through a bumpy period, probably at puberty or in adolescent years when relationships loom large. Interrupted schooling may mean extra study is needed, although many youngsters with Crohn's achieve their full academic potential without any help.

Tilly

Tilly and her brother Nat both developed Crohn's in the same year, although he was ten years older. Nat was 24 and living with his girlfriend when the bouts of diarrhea and vomiting began. Tilly was only 14, and rather fed up. All the other girls were starting their periods and wearing bras, while she remained small and dainty—and childlike. Partly because she was not distracted by an interest in boys, she did particularly well at her studies.

If it had not been for the stomachaches and the increasing bouts of feeling sick and generally unwell and exhausted, one would have expected Tilly to thrive in her high-school years. But by age 16, she was seriously worried about not having started her period and about having hardly any figure. She was still only 4 feet 10 inches tall, and had been that height for ages. No one suspected Crohn's disease at first, but one of the abdominal X-rays provided the first clue.

Tilly was very much into organic and natural foods, so she showed great determination by sticking with the unpalatable elemental diet for weeks, and later a less restricted one that avoided all dairy products. She has done well—with no steroids—and only has to go back on the elemental diet for three or four weeks at a time when the symptoms creep back.

Chapter 5

Patients over Sixty

Crohn's disease is typically a young adults' illness. In fact, it was not until the 1950s, a quarter century after it was recognized and named, that anyone realized that it could affect people who were over 50, let alone those 60 or older. Today, 10 percent of those newly diagnosed with Crohn's are over 50, and include more women than men.

Until very recently, it has been almost impossible to distinguish between Crohn's and the other IBD, ulcerative colitis, in this age group, particularly since Crohn's in the elderly occurs in the colon rather than the ileum. The diagnosis used to be in doubt in up to 20 percent of cases, but this statistic is improving. The symptoms are much the same in both illnesses, and the appearance to the naked eye of the lining of the intestine is similar, with thickening, ulceration, and deep fissures. The advent of the fiber-optic endoscope has made accurate diagnosis feasible. This flexible instrument allows the doctor to see around corners and to take samples of tissue for examination under a microscope. Examination by this method is called endoscopy or, more specifically when done in the colon, *colonoscopy*. It is quite a tricky procedure, however, compared with the older method of passing a shorter, rigid tube called a sigmoidoscope through the anus.

Now that doctors are diagnosing Crohn's disease across the whole age range, it is becoming clear that there are two peaks in the incidence of the disease (*incidence* refers to the number of new cases cropping up each year). The two peak age groups are 20 to 29 and 70 to 79. In the older age group, there is a possibility that another condition, *ischemic colitis*, may be clouding the issue. In older people the little arteries supplying blood to the lining of the large intestine sometimes get furred up. With poor circulation the tissues are subject to ulceration and inflammation, resulting in diarrhea and bleeding. It may be that some people diagnosed as having Crohn's are really suffering from ischemic colitis. Like so much about Crohn's disease, the jury is still out.

People over 60 with Crohn's react differently from younger adults, not in the type of symptoms but in their severity. On the whole, older people fare better.

- They have fewer complaints of bad pain, by about 30 percent.

- There is less likelihood, by 75 percent, of sizeable lumps of inflamed tissue (*granulomas*) developing.

- They have less diarrhea.

- The ileum is 30 percent less likely to be affected.

- The colon—particularly the lower part, the storage section—is more likely to be involved.

- The left side of the abdomen is affected in 40 percent of older sufferers, compared with younger people in whom the right side is nearly always the site of any pain.

One disadvantage of the symptoms being milder in the elderly is that a tendency not to complain, not to "bother the doctor," may result in an unnecessary time lag between the first symptoms and the diagnosis. Valuable time is wasted, with the risk of complications developing, including obstruction and bowel cancer.

THE LEADING SYMPTOMS IN THE ELDERLY

- Diarrhea is the most common symptom but is not usually as severe as in other age groups.

- Loss of weight is the second most common, and since one is less likely to notice clothes getting looser than tighter, a regular weigh-in is good policy.

- Abdominal discomfort, turning into pain, is the third most common symptom.

- Elevated temperature occurs more often than in younger people.

- Copious bleeding from the rectum is typical of the older Crohn's sufferer, with an increased likelihood of anemia as a result.

- The part around the anus—the perianal area—is involved more often than in younger adults, but not as severely as among adolescents (see page 43).

Because the symptoms are often milder in seniors, and because they are apt to assume that they must accept some imperfections of bodily function as they grow older, it can happen that the first time the older person with Crohn's consults the doctor is in an emergency. For instance, the ulceration may have penetrated the wall of the colon and set off peritonitis in the covering membranes. Or acute obstruction of the bowel, particularly the small bowel, may occur. In either of these situations there is severe pain, and often collapse, and the victim must be rushed to the hospital for intensive treatment.

DIVERTICULAR DISEASE

This is a very common wear-and-tear disorder of the colon, affecting 30 percent of patients over 60. The intestinal wall becomes weaker after age 50, like other parts of the body. Weak spots in the colon walls bulge into little pouches called *diverticula*, a condition known as *diverticulosis*. Naturally enough, some of the bowel contents, which have by now become feces, get caught up in the pouches, which may trigger painful inflammation and infection in the gut lining—*diverticulitis*. There may be some bleeding, but not as bad as in Crohn's.

Diverticular disease is unpleasant in its own right, but not dangerous. The big danger is that the doctor may misdiagnose Crohn's as this relatively unimportant condition, delaying proper treatment. To confuse the issue further, Crohn's frequently develops in a part of the colon already affected by diverticular disease.

Philippa

Philippa, aged 66, had always had trouble with her bowels. She had a tendency toward constipation, for which she had taken various laxatives for years. Her doctor believed such a habit predisposed the colon to develop Crohn's disease, cancer, or the much more common, less important diverticular disease. When she was 62 Philippa began to have what was unusual for her—loose stools. She had bouts of diarrhea with blood and mucous, accompanied by abdominal discomfort, just short of pain. Reasonably enough, her doctor assumed she had the common, recurrent condition of infected diverticula—diverticulitis. He prescribed antibiotics, but they did no good. The condition rumbled on.

Good periods alternated with the episodes of diarrhea. Her doctor began to have doubts about the diagnosis and was anxious not to miss a serious illness. He administered a blood test, which showed that Philippa had a hemoglobin level of 7.8 g/dl (grams per deciliter; the normal range for a woman is 11.5–16.5 g/dl), indicating anemia. She also had a low level of albumin (26 g/l instead of 36–47), and a high white blood cell count. These results pointed to active disease and were consistent with Crohn's. The specialist settled the matter with a colonoscopy. Philippa had Crohn's disease. She responded well to medicines for her anemia and her Crohn's disease, respectively, plus a high-protein, high-calorie diet.

It is vitally important to recognize and begin the treatment of Crohn's promptly in the elderly, even more so than in younger adults. Older people are more susceptible to serious complications, such as toxic dilatation of the colon, perforation (a break in the intestinal wall), septicemia (blood poisoning), or severe hemorrhage causing a dangerous drop in the volume of circulating blood. This disrupts the essential working of the heart and lungs (see chapter 6).

CORRECT DIAGNOSIS: POINTS TO LOOK OUT FOR

Crohn's disease is likely to be a long, smoldering illness accompanied by loss of weight, while diverticular disease presents itself in recurrent acute attacks of abdominal pain, without weight loss, and without the general malaise of Crohn's. Bleeding from the rectum is more severe in Crohn's, with anemia a likely result. The symptoms of anemia itself are often vague, but they include weakness, fatigue, shortness of breath, dizziness, headache, tinnitus, insomnia, and swollen ankles.

The other disorder that often gets confused with Crohn's is ischemic colitis. This differs from Crohn's in coming on suddenly, often in a person who already has some heart, blood pressure, or circulatory problem. Bleeding or clotting problems after surgery of any kind are likely in people who are susceptible to ischemic colitis, while the inflammatory lumps of granulomatous tissue characteristic of Crohn's are never present in this disorder.

THE OUTLOOK

The outlook is better for Crohn's patients who are elderly when they contract the disease. They stand only a 42 percent chance of requiring surgery, which is a good deal less than in younger patients and in those suffering from ulcerative colitis. What is most cheering is that the prognosis for seniors with Crohn's has improved enormously over the last few years. This is largely because of earlier, more accurate diagnosis, so that appropriate management is begun sooner. Formerly, even a barium X-ray to show the outline of the colon often revealed only the bulges of diverticular disease, and Crohn's went unrecognized. The use of endoscopy and biopsy (see pages 68 and 69) has put the correct answer beyond doubt.

Treatment also has improved in the life-threatening situations, not so much because of the drugs, but because of better tube feeding or intravenous nourishment; more-sophisticated, modern methods of intensive care; and new, safer surgery. Chapters 8 through 10 describe in detail the medical and surgical treatments. The positive options now available for Crohn's patients are just as effective in older sufferers as in other age groups.

Paul

Paul had retired from his merchant-banking firm nearly ten years before and was concentrating on his golf. He had been the club captain twice. At 70 he had never had a major illness, and his only operation had been for a hernia. Apart from a slight fall-off in energy he felt as good as ever. He occasionally experienced noisy gurgling in his abdomen and mild cramping pains that did not last. So he was unprepared for the night when he woke at 2 A.M., vomited several times, had one bowel movement, and experienced excruciating colicky pains in the middle of his abdomen.

The doctor diagnosed obstruction, and Paul was rushed off to the hospital. His doctor had been right, and the obstruction proved to be due to a stricture (narrowing) in Paul's small intestine near the junction with the caecum. The surgeon removed the affected part and constructed an ileostomy—an opening on the surface of the abdomen—from the healthy part of the ileum. Paul recovered well from the operation and has become good friends with his ileostomy nurse.

He is thinking of trying nine holes very soon.

Chapter 6

Effects outside the Digestive System

You would not guess that a teenager with a painful ankle was exhibiting the first sign of Crohn's disease, or that the lumps that showed up out of the blue on Pat's shins could have anything to do with an illness in her small intestine. Yet they did.

Almost any bodily system can be caught up in the Crohn's process, probably through a poorly understood immunity reaction. These off-the-track symptoms are important not only because they are unpleasant in themselves and require treatment, but because they may alert you or your doctor to the possibility of Crohn's disease. They can make you take notice of any mild bowel symptoms you might have ignored and stimulate your doctor to run some tests.

SKIN DISORDERS

These are the most obvious symptoms. There are three types associated with Crohn's, all with impressive names: *erythema nodosum*, which are the lumps that Pat had (see below), its cousin *erythema multiforme*, and *pyoderma gangrenosum*. Erythema multiforme consists of raised lumps often of a target shape, blistering in the middle, but with no fixed pattern. Pyoderma gangrenosum is the most serious and it only occurs in Crohn's or the other IBD, ulcerative colitis. It begins with a batch of spots, full of pus like boils, which break down to form ulcers. They are caused by a common germ, the staphylococcus, and the first line of treatment is with antibiotics.

Pat

Pat was 29. She often had stomachaches and diarrhea, and the possibility of Crohn's disease or ulcerative colitis had been mentioned but never followed up. Then some painful, dusky, purplish-red lumps appeared on her legs, and she felt ill—as though she had the flu. All her joints ached, she had a fever, and she could not face food. Her doctor recognized the characteristic skin reaction of erythema nodosum and narrowed possible causes to the contraceptive pill, chlamydia, various infections—and IBD.

Pat had to stay in bed for a week, but it was a month before the lumps went down, leaving what looked like bruises that lasted several more weeks. By that time, based on what Pat could tell him, the doctor had worked out that she had IBD. The small dose of a steroid that she was given chased off the skin problem at the same time that it eased the symptoms of her bowel troubles.

ARTHRITIS

Arthritis is the disorder most frequently encountered outside the digestive system in Crohn's disease. Sometimes—in about half the cases—the pain, called *arthralgia*, is present in the joints, but is unaccompanied by any inflammation or any abnormality in an X-ray. The joints most commonly affected are the hips and ankles, perhaps because they are weight-bearing. The sacroiliac joints, which are at the bottom of the back, or the back itself, can also be affected. A particularly disabling back disorder, *ankylosing spondylitis*, can occur with Crohn's, but fortunately it is rare.

Zoe

Zoe was 15, a lanky type, and had recently been complaining

that she was tired. She had a tiny appetite, and everyone thought this was a way to keep slim. While her friends were gradually filling out their bras and getting taller, Zoe was as flat as a board and losing weight. It was all put down to her fussy refusal to eat properly. Her period had not started yet, but a late start was a family trait, so no one was greatly concerned.

Now Zoe started saying that she could not walk because her hip joints hurt. X-rays showed nothing, so she was sent to a child-guidance clinic. She stopped complaining, so perhaps the discussions had helped. It was not until seven months later that the colicky abdominal pains began. This time the investigations included a special type of X-ray with a barium meal, a drink that shows up as it passes down the alimentary canal. This showed the "string sign"—a much narrowed segment of the small intestine, representing an area of spasm in the muscles of its wall and a dead giveaway for Crohn's disease.

With the diagnosis made, Zoe was given the appropriate treatment. After a brief boost with a steroid to start things off, she received a drug called sulfasalazine and as much nourishment as she could manage. The hope is that there is enough growth potential left in her long bones to make up for the period of snail-paced development.

ANEMIA

Anemia is commonplace—practically routine—in Crohn's disease, especially the simple type caused by iron deficiency. If the small intestine is not functioning properly, iron, among other important minerals and vitamins, cannot be absorbed. If, on the other hand, the colon is the part of the gut most affected, bleeding from the ulcerated areas leads to the same result. The body normally recycles its iron so that when red blood corpuscles are discarded, usually when they are about six weeks old, the iron is salvaged for the new replacement cells. When bleeding occurs for any reason the iron is lost together with all the other constituents of the blood.

Another kind of anemia that occurs less often in Crohn's disease is *autoimmune hemolytic anemia*. Autoimmune refers to a mistake made by the immune system so that it attacks and tries to destroy some of its own cells as though they were invaders. In this case it is the red blood cells that are attacked. Hemolytic means blood-destroying. In hemolytic anemia the pigment from the cells is released into the fluid part of the blood, the plasma, and shows up yellowish in the skin, the membranes, and the white part of the eyes. Finally it is absorbed into the urine, making it a darker color than usual.

The faulty working of the immune system that may result in this type of anemia is a poorly understood part of Crohn's. When red blood cells have been destroyed, replacements cannot be manufactured properly if there is a shortage, because of malabsorption, of vitamins B12 and folate. This compounds the situation. There is also the *hypochromic anemia* of chronic diseases in general. The appearance of the blood under the microscope is the same as in iron-deficiency anemia, but the iron stores are there—there just seems to be a block on using them.

The main symptoms of anemia, such as fatigue, pallor, and shortness of breath, are common to all three types.

Colin

Colin Chan left Hong Kong when the city was handed over to China and managed to land a good administrative job in a hospital. He was 32 and had high hopes for his future. The snag was that, ridiculous as it seemed at his age, he was slowing down. Everything took twice as long and seemed such an effort. He huffed when he played tennis and could feel his heart thumping away. He was also having pains in the lower right corner of his abdomen and had lost his appetite. Sometimes he had a throbbing headache—not the tension kind—and although he felt exhausted, he could not sleep. Once or twice he felt quite dizzy and thought he might faint.

When the ringing in his ears started he decided to ask a doctor friend at the hospital to check him over to see whether there was anything wrong, or if he was just a hypochondriac. Colin's friend did not pick up on the slight yellowing of the whites of his eyes and skin, nor did he ask about the color of his urine, so jaundice did not figure in his mind. However, he did arrange a blood test and found that Colin had a mix of two kinds of anemia. He had deficiencies of iron, and of the vitamins B12 and folic acid.

Then the young doctor homed in on the two symptoms that were not caused by anemia: the pain in the appendix area and the loss of appetite. The complete picture emerged: Crohn's disease causing malabsorption, in turn causing anemia. Colin required dietary supplements, and he also had a stricturoplasty, a repair of a diseased part of the ileum that was in danger of blockage. Azathioprine was the nonsteroidal medication chosen to control the Crohn's after that.

Colin exhibited a number of the usual symptoms of anemia, but fortunately missed out on chest pains (*angina*), swollen ankles (*edema*), poor vision, an elevated heart rate, and the feeling of pins and needles in the fingers and toes.

EYE DISORDERS

Inflammation of the eye is another unexpected problem accompanying Crohn's disease. Any part of the eye may be affected.

Stephen

Stephen blamed the sore, gritty feeling in his eyes on staring at a computer screen so much of the time. He had conjunctivitis, inflammation of the "skin" covering the front of the eye. His Crohn's disease had been in remission for several months, but he had recently undergone a very stressful period at work, with a new boss who wanted everything done differently. The conjunctivitis was the first indication of a relapse, accompanied by more frequent bowel movements and a mild fever in the evenings. An increase in Stephen's medication and a few sessions of counseling helped to avert a more serious attack.

Conjunctivitis like Stephen's is the simplest and least serious eye disorder that may be associated with Crohn's disease. Others include *uveitis*, *episcleritis*, *keratitis*, *retinitis*, and *retrobulbar neuritis*—each being inflammation in one or another part of the eye. Any discomfort in the eyes or impairment of vision needs expert attention but also serves as a reminder to the patient with established Crohn's disease to review his or her current treatment and lifestyle.

HEART AND BLOOD VESSELS

The heart and blood vessels may seem far-removed from intestinal illness, but any blood vessel, from the big arteries and veins down to the tiniest capillaries, may react to Crohn's disease (and some other chronic conditions) by inflammation. This is called *vasculitis*. One theory holds that vasculitis of the small vessels in the gut wall underlies the tendency to ulceration. Some people with Crohn's develop *pericarditis* or *myocarditis*, inflammation of the membrane enclosing the heart or of the heart muscle itself, respectively. The symptoms are chest pain, shortness of breath, and fainting spells.

LIVER AND GALL BLADDER

A number of problems under this heading may be an indirect result of Crohn's disease. Cholesterol gallstones are common, but especially in Crohn's, from middle age onward. They only cause trouble if a stone gets wedged in the bile duct, which can set off inflammation of the whole gall bladder/bile duct system.

Aaron

Aaron was 53. He had coped with Crohn's disease for eight years and felt he had it beaten when he was woken up out of the blue at 2 A.M. by an agonizingly sharp pain in his upper abdomen. He thought it was due to a cholesterol-rich birthday dinner he had enjoyed with his family that evening. The meal had featured goulash and a luscious creamy dessert and may indeed have stimulated extra activity in the digestive system.

The pain was not colicky, but continued at full strength all the time. When the doctor arrived, bleary-eyed, it had shifted slightly to the right and even Aaron's shoulder hurt on that side. Then he started vomiting and his temperature skyrocketed. In the hospital, X-rays and ultrasound showed gallstones. Aaron was given a morphine injection for the pain and an IV to increase his fluid level. When the acute symptoms settled, the question of surgery came up. The Crohn's was no bar to that, and his gall bladder, with the stones it contained, was successfully removed.

A much rarer disorder is *sclerosing cholangitis*, an inflammation of the bile duct with narrowing from scar tissue, much like stricture formation in Crohn's ileitis (inflammation of the ileum). Cholangitis nearly always arises in Crohn's disease and ulcerative colitis, the other IBD. It does not come on suddenly like gallstone pain, but shows up first with jaundice and fever that come and go, and pain in the same area as gall bladder pain. Often the skin itches all over. Antibiotics help, but steroids are no use.

Cirrhosis of the liver has a reputation for being associated with alcohol, and it often is, but teetotaller Crohn's patients can also develop it. The liver, in the upper right abdomen, at first enlarges with fat, then shrinks and becomes knobby as scar tissue forms. Cirrhosis is more dangerous than Crohn's disease.

Gordon

Gordon was 34. He had had Crohn's since age 19. His work as a freelance journalist meant that many of the best assignments seemed to be handed out in bars, not that he was a heavy drinker, unlike some of his colleagues. Gradually Gordon was becoming aware of vague discomfort in his upper abdomen, different from the pain low down on the right that he felt when his Crohn's was acting up. Otherwise there was nothing that the Crohn's might not account for: tiredness, weakness, loss of appetite with nausea, bloating, and loss of weight. There was nothing specific about any of these symptoms.

Only after he fell off his motorcycle did he have a chat with his doctor. Gordon had not suffered any bone injury, but he did incur extensive bruising. He told the doctor as a matter of interest that he bruised very easily these days and mentioned that he "hadn't been feeling too great," what with the discomfort in his abdomen. The doctor found a place that was tender when he pressed it, under Gordon's ribs on the right, and he ran a few blood tests. They showed that his liver was not functioning properly, possibly the beginning of cirrhosis. Some of Gordon's journalist friends had come to grief that way, so he was scared enough to take it seriously when told that he must give up alcohol altogether if he wanted to live a long life.

Since he was not addicted, Gordon was able to stick to the plan, and he also followed—under advice—a totally rearranged diet: low in fat but high in protein and carbohydrate, with supplements of the vitamins B12, C, D, and folic acid, and of calcium. After three months his liver-function tests were near normal. Fatty liver—the final diagnosis—is fairly common in Crohn's but is reversible with strict attention to diet and a lifestyle without alcohol.

URINARY SYSTEM

The urinary system is no more immune than other parts of the body from the effects of Crohn's disease. Sometimes one of the swollen parts of the ileum may press on one of the ureters, the twin tubes that convey urine from the kidneys to the bladder. If the urine cannot flow down freely on one side there is back pressure on that kidney, causing pain in the small of the back. A danger of infection results, accompanied by sudden pain in the loin and radiating around to the front, vomiting, and high fever. Antibiotic treatment is urgently required.

Edmund had a very different urinary problem.

Edmund

Edmund had been a Crohn's sufferer for six years and had managed fairly well with several medicines. He was 39 when he started having bladder infections, one after another—fairly unusual for a man. Antibiotics helped, but not for long; it was a miserable situation. What took him by surprise was that he seemed to be passing bubbles of air in his urine. When it happened again his doctor referred him to a urogenital surgeon. Examination with a cystoscope, an instrument for looking inside the bladder, provided the answer—a fistula coming through from the colon. An operation was required to remove the offending piece of colon, ulcerated through by Crohn's, and the bladder was repaired. It healed within two weeks and Edmund has had no urinary infections since. No bladder could have stood up to a constant leakage of material from the colon.

One residual problem was Edmund's dip into depression, with low moods, poor sleep and loss of appetite. With Crohn's he could not afford to lose any more weight, so after he left the surgical ward, he spent six weeks as a day patient in the psychiatric department. His treatment involved a mix of individual cognitive therapy, various group therapies, including one for drama, and an antidepressant. The combination worked, both mentally and physically.

THE RESPIRATORY SYSTEM

The respiratory system is affected in as many as 30 percent of Crohn's disease cases, but usually the symptoms are too mild to be troublesome. The lung may react to Crohn's with what is called *alveolitis*, an inflammation of the small, delicate air sacs that comprise the lung tissue. If a significant number are involved the patient may develop a persistent, dry cough and become short of breath while exercising.

A chest X-ray will reveal the problem, and treatment is much the same as for Crohn's itself: the steroid prednisolone backed up by azathioprine, to reduce the need for a large dose of the steroid.

METASTATIC CROHN'S DISEASE

All the conditions described so far as linked with Crohn's disease but outside the digestive system arise as a reaction to the intestinal illness in one way or another. Metastatic Crohn's disease is different. It *is* Crohn's disease. Patches of typical Crohn's inflammation appear somewhere unconnected with any other affected area—it is not a matter of simple spread. Any part of the skin may show Crohn's-type swelling, redness, and ulceration, but most often it is below the waist, for instance at the navel or on the thigh. The genitals and the skin between them and the anus are quite often involved.

One young fellow accepted his Crohn's with good grace until a strange sore place appeared on his penis. He went to the clinic, furiously thinking that his trusted partner had infected him with an STD (sexually transmitted disease). None of the usual infections in that area were responsible, but a sample (biopsy) of the skin showed unmistakable Crohn's and a few ordinary skin bacteria. Fortunately, the sore patch responded to a steroid cream.

Of course not every Crohn's patient may experience all or even any of the unpleasant symptoms cataloged in this chapter. However, it is helpful to be aware of them and to realize that they could be connected with Crohn's disease so that the patient and his or her health-care professionals when exploring treatment options are optimally equipped to restore the patient to a full life.

Chapter 7

Proper Diagnosis: The Full Range of Tests

You have symptoms you want to be rid of, and they could be caused by Crohn's disease—or one of several other disorders. Before any treatment can begin, your doctor needs to find out for sure which one it is.

To start the diagnostic hunt he or she will want to hear about the information your body itself is providing in the form of symptoms, such as pain, loose stools, and weight loss. How long have you had them, and have you any idea what triggered them? Have you experienced anything similar before, and if so, what happened? If any of your relatives have had bowel problems, what was the diagnosis?

The physical examination may reveal a tender place in the appendix area, and your doctor may be able to feel a definite lump of inflamed tissue. He or she will also be able to judge if you have recently lost weight and whether you have the general pallor of skin and membranes that indicates anemia.

After the physical examination and all the questions, you will probably be asked to provide a stool sample. A pale, frothy stool indicates malabsorption, evidence that your small intestine is not working properly. Blood and mucous in the sample indicates that the colon is inflamed and ulcerated, but if bleeding occurs in the small intestine, which is less common, the stool is black and tarry.

Part of the specimen will be sent to the laboratory for culture, to find what bacteria will grow and to test which antibiotics are effective against them. There will be a heavier growth of bacteria than normal in Crohn's, but unfortunately the chief suspect, Mycobacterium paratuberculosis (Mptb for short), is extremely slow and difficult to grow in culture. In a recent research study it took between 13 and 40 months. This is obviously no help in diagnosing what is wrong with someone who is suffering today.

Identifying the particular mycobacterium has also presented major problems, but the development of DNA probes promises useful results (see chapter 15).

Another big snag is that the abdomen keeps its secrets hidden. You cannot tell from the outside what is going on inside any more than you can tell by looking at the outside of someone's house what they are doing inside. Fortunately, technology has brought some of the secrets of abdominal disorders out of the realms of guesswork. A whole range of tests is now available for detecting and assessing Crohn's disease.

RADIOLOGY

X-rays were first used in the investigation of Crohn's in 1934, only two years after it was recognized as an illness. The intestines do not show up in X-rays, so they need to be outlined by a material that is opaque to them. A suspension of barium is harmless and shows up well. It is routinely used in so-called barium "meals" and enemas. An extra refinement is to introduce air or gas into the part to be visualized. In X-rays this appears black in contrast to the white produced by barium, and the combination is called *double-contrast radiology*.

Barium Meal and Follow-Through

Before you begin you need to have your stomach and intestines empty—a matter of fasting, as for surgery—but the examination requires only outpatient attendance. The meal consists of a glass of white liquid, usually flavored with peppermint. You swallow it slowly, and the progress of the barium is tracked by X-ray as it moves down the alimentary tract. While this method is still in use, it has been superseded by enteroclysis (see below) in some centers.

Enteroclysis

An improvement on the barium-meal method, because it provides more and clearer detail, is the infusion of the suspension of barium directly into the intestine through a tube. This is called *enteroclysis*.

Even the tiny aphthoid ulcers in the lining of the gut can be seen with this method. Crops of these in the small intestine are probably the first visible sign of Crohn's. Larger ulcers develop later, with the general thickening of the gut wall. Greatly narrowed segments, the "string sign," are especially characteristic of the disease. They are caused by spasm of the gut muscles. Cobblestone patterning occurs only in severe Crohn's. An irregular arrangement of patches of inflammation is another strong indication of Crohn's. "Skip" lesions are patches like islands of inflammation in a sea of normal tissue, as though the disease had missed or skipped some areas. All or some of these may be recognizable in a barium X-ray and support a diagnosis of Crohn's affecting the small intestine.

An interesting and characteristic effect of malabsorption is the clumping of the barium suspension in the ileum, caused by an excess of digestive juices.

These X-rays may also pick up some common complications— sinuses and fistulas. Sinuses are ulcerated tracks that go through the full thickness of the gut wall, while in fistulas the ulceration extends into some other organ. Barium X-rays, particularly those from enteroclysis in expert hands, give valuable information for diagnosis and pinpointing the site of the problem when surgery is contemplated for obstruction or a fistula.

Howard

Howard was 24 when he started a new job in sales for a company making scientific instruments. He spent a lot of his day traveling from one laboratory to another. He felt perfectly well, aside from the inconvenience of having to find the restroom so often, for his bowels. He also felt a bit tired—and had lost weight. His home was in one of the most beautiful counties in England, and his local hospital was friendly and welcoming. The physician whom Howard saw there suspected Crohn's disease as soon as he heard Howard's story, and he suggested a barium meal and follow-through right away.

Howard found the experience not unpleasant—and very interesting, especially when the doctor explained the relevant X-rays to him. He showed Howard two features that pointed directly to Crohn's—the "string" sign of a very narrow segment of gut, and the flocculation (or clumping) of the barium. Patches of swollen mucous membrane could also be detected in the small intestine, and a few in the first part of the colon.

Howard's Crohn's was mild. He took ten days off work for rest and treatment. Then, with some rearrangement of his work schedule to allow for reasonable breaks and a reengineering of his diet, he remained well—and needed only a nonsteroidal medicine.

Barium Enema

The large intestine is best investigated by a barium enema. This is like any other enema except for the preliminaries. First there is the ordinary examination of the rectal passage with a gloved finger, then a *sigmoidoscopy*, usually a few days before the enema. Since the bowel must be clean and clear for this special enema, the patient is given laxatives and a cleansing wash. Finally the patient is ready for the barium enema, often used in conjunction with air to stretch the colon lining for a better picture. The enema itself, including taking X-rays, takes only 25 to 30 minutes, but older people and those with heart complaints sometimes find the whole procedure rather exhausting. Patients should plan to rest afterwards.

CT Scanning (Computerized Tomography)

This is a different kind of X-ray. It provides a series of shadow pictures of the body as though it was cut in slices one centimeter apart. The big advantage is that the organs surrounding the intestine can also be seen. CT scans are particularly valuable for Crohn's affecting the lowest parts of the alimentary tract—the rectum and around the anus—as barium enemas and follow-throughs do not provide a comprehensible picture in this area.

CT scans are of great help to surgeons in "fistula mapping," where it is essential to know the way the muscles and other organs lie in relation to an ulcerated part. They have a 90 percent success rate in detecting fistulas involving the bladder (see Edmund, page 62).

ENDOSCOPY

Endoscopy means "looking inside" and is the second most frequently used test for Crohn's. The oldest and simplest method is sigmoidoscopy, in which an instrument with a light at the end, the sigmoidoscope, is inserted through the anus into the rectum. It may be a rigid tube, or more recently, a flexible type. It gives a good view of the rectum and sometimes detects an inflamed, ulcerated area that may be missed in a barium enema. It is an advantage for the doctor actually to see the lining of the intestine as opposed to mere outlines and shadows.

Colonoscopy and Ileocolonoscopy

With the wonderful advances in fiber-optic technology, it is now possible to see the full length of the colon, to the caecum, with a colonoscope, and even further, into the ileum—a procedure called *ileocolonoscopy*. The trick of fiber-optics is that whatever the instrument can "see" at its tip is conveyed along the fibers, however long and tortuous their course through the intestines. It grants us the gift of seeing around corners.

The doctor is looking out for:

- Redness and perhaps bleeding from the lining membrane.

- Cobblestoning—the rough, irregular, knobby pattern made by deep cracks dividing up the swollen, edematous tissue (see Daniel, page 38).

- Ulcers—they may be tiny, white, pinhead aphthoid ulcers, with a red base; the deep, punched-out type, sometimes likened to a well; "railroad track" ulcers running in straight lines; or the serpiginous kind in all sorts of shapes.

- Stenosis—narrowing from any cause. The ileocolonoscope can be slim enough to be passed gently into the narrow part to discover whether it has a generally swollen or lumpy lining, or if tough, fibrous scarring is constricting the passage—or if something outside the intestine is pressing on it.

- Pseudopolyps—small tags of inflamed, swollen lining membrane protruding like fingers. Usually they are unmistakable, but if there is any doubt that they may be true polyps, a biopsy is easily done.

Another brilliant facility of the fiber-optic endoscope is that it can take minute samples of tissue—biopsies—for microscopical examination. You can imagine how useful and reassuring it can be to be able to check that an odd, lumpy mass is not cancer but Crohn's.

Colonoscopy and ileocolonoscopy are the top-notch test methods in Crohn's, requiring a high degree of skill and experience, and they are usually available only in specialized centers. Barium X-rays are a trustworthy fallback if you find yourself far from a big city.

Other types of endoscopy are used in other areas. If you have symptoms relating to your stomach or duodenum, *gastroscopy* or *duodenoscopy*, respectively, are the standard means for assessing the situation. On the rare occasions when the esophagus seems to be the site of Crohn's symptoms, a simple, rigid *esophagoscope* can be slipped in. A mild, muscle-relaxant sedative, like diazepam, takes the edge off any anxiety and discomfort during these procedures.

ULTRASOUND AND ENDOSONOGRAPHY

Ultrasound is another form of investigation, most familiar from its routine use in pregnancy. Inaudible (to us) sound waves are directed toward the part to be examined and are measured as they bounce back, or echo, producing a black-and-white image. The whole process is filmed, with stills taken as necessary. Endosonography entails that for greater precision the *echoprobe* that emits and picks up the sound waves is put inside the rectum.

Endosonography (ES) is most useful when there is an abscess or a fistula in the pelvic area that is particularly difficult to "see" by other methods. It is important to know the exact location of either of these complications in relation to other vital structures in this crowded area before active treatment is begun. ES is also employed to check the results of medical or surgical treatment before deciding on the next step. It is ideal to try simple rest and medicines first and check whether this treatment is working before launching into complex surgery in a sensitive area.

Dorothy

Dorothy felt ill. She was 47 and had been on a roller coaster of relapse and recovery for two years. Her Crohn's had come on originally when she was about 30, and although she had endured two or three bouts of illness she had always bounced back quite quickly. This time she continued to have a dragging pain in her pelvis and persistent fever. Passing a stool was agony.

Sigmoidoscopy and colonoscopy were not helpful, but echosonography with the scope in the vagina showed a cavity that did not produce an echo. It was an abscess, positioned too low to have shown up in the other tests. Dorothy was not keen on surgery, so she was treated medically. After three months another endosonograph showed that the abscess was definitely smaller, and by ten months it could no longer be seen. And Dorothy felt well.

RADIO-LABELED LEUKOCYTE SCANNING

Leukocytes are the white cells in the blood. Their major function is fighting infection; they are the foot soldiers in the battle, so many thousands are needed, including reserves that can be called upon when there is illness. They are transported in the bloodstream and, like passengers on a bus, stop off at the appropriate places.

In a radio-labeled leukocyte scan a blood sample is taken from a vein. The white cells in it are "labeled" with a short-life radioactive tag, and then returned to circulation. Their progress can be followed with a gamma camera, which "photographs" radiation. The white cells congregate in trouble spots within a few hours, pointing out areas of inflammation in both the small and large intestines. The advantages of this kind of scanning are that it involves no risks, no special preparation, and no more discomfort than two pinpricks, one to withdraw and one to return the blood sample. It can be used safely in someone who is severely ill and for whom colonoscopy or ileocolonoscopy would be dangerous.

Radio-labeled leukocyte scanning has been proved a more sensitive test for IBD than barium examinations, and it provides a valuable objective assessment of how effective a particular treatment has been. It is at the forefront of modern investigative techniques, and further research is actively taking place as you read.

LABORATORY TESTS

Crohn's disease is an illness that fluctuates from the acute and incapacitating at one time to almost complete remission at another. It is useful to have some pointers to what is going on in the background. If you are in a bad phase, is it beginning to get better—or worse? If the illness is quiescent, what is the likelihood of relapse? Such considerations are particularly relevant if you are going through a period of emotional strain. Laboratory tests give your doctor factual information on which to base an anti-Crohn's strategy. It is helpful to have some idea what the results mean.

Active Inflammation

This is reflected by testing for two conditions:

- The ESR (erythrocyte sedimentation rate) is higher than the normal 0–6 mm (millimeters) per hour when there is infection or inflammation. More than 20 mm per hour shows a severe condition.

- The number of white blood cells (leukocytes) in your blood is above the normal 4,000–11,000 per microliter (leukocytosis).

Anemia

If you are anemic the hemoglobin level in your blood is reduced. Normal levels are:

- 130–180 g/l (grams per liter) for a man
- 115–165 g/l for a woman

Malabsorption

This is the result of the small intestine being unable to function properly. It may manifest in a shortage of certain minerals in your blood. The normal ranges are:

- calcium: 2.12–2.62 mmol/l (millimoles per liter)
- magnesium: 0.75–1 mmol/l
- iron: 14–32 micromol/l (micromols per liter) for a man; 10–28 micromol/l for a woman
- zinc: 8–29 micromol/l

Other substances that may be inadequately absorbed in Crohn's (and their normal ranges) are:

- vitamin B12: 160–925 nanograms/l (nanograms per liter; B12 is lacking in some forms of anemia)
- folate: 6–21 micrograms/l (micrograms per liter; lacking in some forms of anemia)

- albumin: 37–47 g/l (grams per liter; albumin, or protein in the blood, is low in Crohn's sufferers because of poor absorption of proteins in general)

Special Tests for Malabsorption

- Fats: if these are not being absorbed properly from the ileum, the stool will contain more than 7 grams of fat in 24 hours.

- Carbohydrates: lactose-tolerance test and hydrogen breath test.

Evelyn

Evelyn, at 28, was engaged to be married. Like all Crohn's sufferers in her situation, she worried about the sexual aspect. Suppose she was seized with uncontrollable diarrhea at the critical moment, or one of her occasional periods of feverishness coincided with the honeymoon? They always seemed to come when she was anxious.

In the days preceding the wedding Evelyn's abdomen was a little tender and she was passing two or three bowel movements a day. She tried to tell herself that it was only tension. Then her temperature began sneaking up to 101°F in the evenings. The doctor checked for active disease with an ESR and a blood count. They were both slightly out of the normal range. Evelyn asked if there was any way at this stage to ward off what seemed a mild—so far—threat of relapse. The doctor temporarily added a small dose of methylprednisolone to her nonsteroidal medication, but gave no promises. However, Evelyn sailed through the wedding and the honeymoon without mishap, and when she returned, had a checkup. Her elevated ESR and leukocytosis (excess of white cells) had subsided.

TESTS IN PRACTICE

The main point of tests is to find out what is causing the unwelcome symptoms. Since different conditions require different kinds of treatment, it is important to get the answer right. The steps toward reaching a diagnosis begin with the patient's complaints and may end with the ultimate: ileocolonoscopy and serial biopsies, with laboratory tests and X-rays en route. But no single test is 100 percent reliable.

Wendy

Wendy was 16 and in the middle of final exams when a cramping pain in her abdomen doubled her up. A minute later she was running to the bathroom with diarrhea. The cramps and the diarrhea, which poured out like water, persisted and Wendy felt sick and dizzy. No way could she continue with the exam, so the teacher sent her home in a taxi. She only vomited once, but she felt alternately boiling hot and freezing cold. When her mother came home from work she found Wendy in bed with all her clothes on and a temperature of 106°F.

The doctor took a sample of the watery stool for culture and advised Wendy to drink as much as possible in the form of fruit-flavored drinks and tea rather than plain water. He prescribed loperamide to control the diarrhea, but no antibiotics at this stage, since they could make matters worse. The symptoms were slow to settle, and since the culture showed the presence of salmonella, he gave her some ciprofloxacillin, which is particularly effective against this infection. Even so, Wendy continued to have pain in her lower abdomen and to pass three or four bowel movements a day.

An ileocolonoscopy showed shallow ulcers with red, inflamed edges in the lining of the colon on the left, and a cluster of aphthoid ulcers on the right. Under the microscope a small collection of granuloma cells could be seen. All of this was consistent with Crohn's disease, and at this point the diagnosis lay between this and salmonella colitis.

Six months later, a repeat ileocolonoscopy showed that all the ulcers had healed and both ileum and colon were clear. The microscopic appearances had reverted to normal, too. Crohn's disease was ruled out, and the final diagnosis was acute salmonella colitis, from which Wendy had recovered.

Martin

Martin was 18 when he went on vacation to Turkey, where he had an attack of traveler's diarrhea. At least that was what he thought. It started with twinges of pain in the appendix area, mild nausea, and colic. When the diarrhea started he went to a local pharmacist, who suggested paregoric to calm his bowels down. Since he was due to go home in a day or two, he decided to see his own doctor as soon as he got back. He was still having colicky pains and episodes of painful straining to pass small stools, streaked with blood and pus. The culture, when the result came back, showed a bug called shigelli flexneri, often a cause of dysentery. After a course of the appropriate antibiotic, Martin's symptoms began to subside, but within a few days they all came back, so an ileocolonoscopy was performed.

The operator saw that Martin's colon was inflamed and had some shallow ulcers throughout its length; biopsies confirmed this. Martin's illness was labeled acute self-limited colitis—but it did not self-limit. It went on. Six months later, the doctor had to accept that Martin had chronic inflammatory bowel disease—probably Crohn's.

Even microscopical examination of a sample of the gut lining cannot provide an ironclad guarantee of the correct diagnosis. Various intestinal infections can mimic IBD of the colon, but they do not affect the ileum, except possibly the last inch or so, where small and large intestine join.

In both these cases it was not until many months after the onset of the symptoms that the diagnosis could be made with certainty. Fortunately, with all the technical help available, such cases are exceptional.

Chapter 8

Treatment Options: Medicines

Crohn's disease is not an illness you simply have to put up with—a range of treatments exists, and at different times you may need more than one of them:

- medicines

- surgery

- diet

- change in lifestyle

- psychological help

Whether you are feeling generally out-of-sorts or you have troublesome symptoms such as pain or diarrhea, your first thought is likely to be, What can I take to make it better? First aid for abdominal pain is a hot-water bottle or the equivalent, and for diarrhea there are several simple over-the-counter medicines that are worth trying:

- Diphenoxylate (Lomotil): two 2.5 mg tablets, three times a day.

- Loperamide (Imodium, Loperagen): 2 mg tablet three times a day.

- Opiate-based antidiarrheals, most commonly paregoric, are sold over the counter as controlled substances in some states. The pharmacist can recommend the dosage.

None of these will be more than a stopgap if you have Crohn's.

STEROIDS

The linchpin in the treatment of Crohn's is the use of steroid medicines—corticosteroids to be exact. Hydrocortisone is the steroid your body makes for itself, in the two small adrenal glands that lie next to the kidneys. As medicines we have a wide range of synthetic steroids, with *prednisolone* the most commonly used.

In the 1950s steroids were being tested on several puzzling illnesses, ulcerative colitis among them. Since they proved helpful in that disorder it was an obvious step to try them in Crohn's. They have proved themselves the most effective and rapidly acting drug treatment available, both in desperately serious situations and where there is chronic active disease grumbling along.

Severe, Acute Illness

In the situation, when your life is on the line, high doses of prednisolone can be injected directly into your veins. If your condition is not critical this treatment can be continued for up to five days, but then if you are not much improved it is time for the other option, surgery, to be used.

All steroids carry the risk of side effects, and these may be dangerous if high doses of steroids are continued for long.

Moderately Severe, Acute Illness

In this much more common situation, the patient is not desperately ill but has several symptoms, such as an elevated temperature accompanied by loss of appetite, pain in the abdomen, diarrhea— and perhaps one of the autoimmune reactions such as conjunctivitis or erythema nodosum (see pages 58–59 and 54).

Effective treatment is certainly called for in such cases. A reasonable regimen would be prednisolone in 5 mg tablets, totaling 20–60 mg daily in water, divided into four doses, for one to two weeks; then gradually reduced to 10–20 mg daily for four to six weeks; then tapered off and stopped.

Chronic Active Illness

Here the symptoms are mild, or die down only to return each time you stop the medication. To suppress the symptoms you will probably need to take prednisolone tablets for an indefinite period in the following dosage: 10–15 mg daily at breakfast time, or 20–30 mg on alternate days, to lessen the risk of tiresome side effects.

Risks

Steroids are wonderful in the way they relieve your symptoms immediately, but there is a price to pay. You must treat them with respect. Risky situations to look out for if you are starting on a steroid include:

- Infections, for instance influenza, tonsillitis, cystitis, or tuberculosis, whether caused by a virus, bacteria, or fungus. The steroid suppresses the body's normal reactions for dealing with the illness.

- Contact with anyone with chicken pox or shingles while on steroids and for three months afterwards. If you are exposed to either of these illnesses, tell your doctor, as you will need immunoglobulin treatment at once and special monitoring. If you develop chicken pox you will need specialist care.

- Recent surgery or accidental injury.

- Recent peptic ulcer, even if it has healed.

- Diabetes, underactive thyroid, or kidney or liver disorder.

- Osteoporosis.

- Glaucoma.

- Pregnancy or breastfeeding.

- Serious psychiatric illness.

- Stressful circumstances.

With children and the elderly you need to be especially aware of any new symptom or change and tell the doctor.

Interactions

You may already be taking some other medicines. Check that they will not clash with the steroid. Beware of interactions with:

- antiepileptics
- blood pressure and heart medicines
- anti-inflammatories, for instance for arthritis
- rifampicin and other drugs for tuberculosis
- antifungals, for instance for thrush
- diuretics
- tablets used for diabetes
- erythromycin (an antibiotic), amphotericin
- salicylates, such as aspirin
- estrogen, as in the contraceptive pill and hormone replacement therapy
- anticoagulants (which prevent clotting)

Main Side Effects

- elevated blood pressure, possibly leading to a heart attack
- water retention
- osteoporosis
- peptic ulcer
- moon face
- florid, red cheeks
- increased facial hair
- acne
- increased weight: fat body on thin legs—"like a lemon on a toothpick"
- backache

- easy bruising, slow healing
- stretch marks on abdomen, bottom, and thighs
- thinning of the skin
- muscle weakness
- impaired fertility
- depression—or the opposite, euphoria—with no cause
- in children, growth slowed down or halted

Dosage

Obviously, with all these unpleasant possible side effects, it makes sense to try to use the smallest effective dose of steroid. It is preferable to take the dose in the morning and every other day. It is safest to receive a tiny regular dose (or none at all), and to have a brief boost only when the illness becomes active. There is no evidence that a small continuous dose of steroid keeps you "safe" during a remission; the on-off system is recommended.

Since the symptoms clear up so well with steroid medicine, you may, naturally, feel that it is doing you good and curing the illness. Steroids have no effect on the course of the illness, but suppress your body's reactions to it, which comprise the symptoms.

Remember that you must not stop your steroid medication suddenly, but withdraw gradually over several weeks.

Topical Steroids

Topical means that they are not taken into your bloodstream but are applied to the affected areas only, thus the danger of side effects is greatly reduced. Steroids are very effective locally, as is demonstrated in skin disorders, but with Crohn's disease the affected parts may be difficult to access, for instance, the small intestine.

Suppositories: Suppositories of steroid may be useful when the rectum is affected.

Enemas: Retention enemas are used in the treatment of Crohn's colitis, but the sensitive rectum may not let you hold the enema long enough to do any good.

Foam enemas are easier to retain and feel pleasanter, but only reach into the rectum.

A special form of prednisolone is used for enemas. However, if enemas are used very often, too much of the steroid is absorbed and there may be side effects.

Infusions: Infusions, or slow drips of steroid into the rectum, are another method of treating the lower part of the intestines.

Poorly Absorbed Steroids

For maximum benefit, steroid medicines taken by mouth are meant to be absorbed into the bloodstream as completely as possible. When a topical effect is required without a high risk of side effects, such as with steroid enemas, a preparation that is not well absorbed but remains on the surface of the tissues is wanted. The most suitable steroids for this purpose include budesonide (used more in the U.K. than the United States) and a special form of prednisolone.

Betamethasone (Diprolene), a favorite steroid in France, is very effective, but because it is well absorbed, tends to cause side effects.

Reactions to Steroids

Not everybody finds steroids helpful. Crohn's patients typically react to them in three ways:

1. Resistance—the symptoms show no improvement.

2. Dependency—the patient starts off with a good response but the symptoms return as soon as steroid treatment is stopped.

3. Prolonged response—the desired result, occurring in over half those who take steroid medicines for Crohn's. The symptoms are suppressed and do not return for at least a month after the steroid is stopped.

The best results are seen in people whose Crohn's affects only the colon, or the colon and ileum, rather than the ileum alone.

Emma

Emma was upset. These things matter when you are 23 and have a reputation as a head-turner. Something disastrous had happened to her face and her figure. Her cheeks were too red and pudgy—"like a hamster," she said. And as for her figure! Her arms and legs were like sticks but her jeans and skirts simply would not fasten: her waist had disappeared. The doctor knew what it was at once.

A few months before, Emma had lost her appetite and a lot of weight—without trying—and had a permanent stomachache. Then the diarrhea began and a funny rash appeared on her legs. She was diagnosed as having Crohn's disease and started on prednisolone. It worked like a charm, but when she stopped treatment a few weeks later the symptoms bounced right back. Emma had gotten back on the steroid for another two months when she noticed these unwelcome changes in her appearance. They were the side effects of the medication. The doctor reduced the dose gradually and then changed the prednisolone to sulfasalazine, a nonsteroid. This kept her symptoms under control, and her face and shape returned to normal.

Most of the other medicines used in Crohn's are aimed at replacing, if only temporarily, the powerful steroids and their side effects, or at least enabling the patient to get by with a lower dose.

SALICYLATE GROUP

Sulfasalazine

Sulfasalazine (Azulfidine) and its modern relatives are the most frequently prescribed medicines in Crohn's disease. Sulfasalazine consists of two drugs: an anti-inflammatory related to aspirin, and an antibacterial, sulfapyridine. It was tailored for the treatment of rheumatoid arthritis but turned out to be disappointing. The bonus for Dr. Nana Swartz was that some of her rheumatoid patients who were also suffering from diarrhea found their bowel symptoms improved considerably, and she reported this finding to the medical press.

While it does not control the acute symptoms of Crohn's as swiftly and dramatically as a steroid, sulfasalazine is efficacious in mild to moderate exacerbations of the illness and for maintenance therapy in periods of quiescence. Applied directly to an inflamed area it is at least as effective as a steroid, so it is useful in rectal disease as an enema. Taken orally, however, it is quickly absorbed high up in the alimentary system, so there is hardly any left to treat the lining of the ileum.

Dosage

- 2–4 tablets (500 mg each) four times a day during an attack
- 4 tablets a day for maintenance

Children over two years should take reduced doses, according to their weight. Sulfasalazine is supplied in tablets, suppositories, a lemon-flavored suspension, and as an enema.

Extra Care: While there are no absolute contraindications, patients and their doctors should be particularly alert to any new or unexplained symptoms if the patient is of retirement age, pregnant or breastfeeding, or has had kidney problems. Warning signs that the drug is not suitable for a particular individual include unexplained bleeding, spontaneous bruising, sore throat, or general malaise. Such patients need a blood test promptly to check that blood is being manufactured normally; a blood dyscrasia—when abnormal blood cells are produced, affecting the whole metabolism—is a rare but dangerous reaction.

Interactions: Interactions may occur with other drugs: digoxin, folate, lactulose—the patient should make sure not to take any of these while on sulfasalazine treatment.

Side Effects

- loss of appetite

- nausea

- headaches

- blood dyscrasia (see above)

- kidney problems

- hair loss

- feelings of pins and needles

- low sperm count

A third of those taking sulfasalazine suffer some side effects.

Mesalamine (Pentasa)

This drug does not include the sulfapyridine component of sulfasalazine, so the side effects are fewer, and it has no deleterious effect on the sperm count. It is particularly recommended for the other IBD, ulcerative colitis, but is less useful in Crohn's affecting only the small intestine. Nevertheless, it is replacing sulfasalazine as the most popular salicylate for treating Crohn's.

Olsalazine (Dipentum)

This medicine is not released in the small intestine, so it is useful only in Crohn's of the colon. Side effects are uncommon apart from diarrhea, which occurs in 6 percent of users, who may have this symptom already. A plus is that not only is the drug harmless to sperm, it is also said to reverse any damage done previously by sulfasalazine.

ANTIBIOTICS

Metronidazole (Flagyl)

Metronidazole is another drug that was developed for a different illness and found to be useful in some cases of Crohn's. It is a first-line antibacterial agent for those organisms that thrive in the air-less depths of the body, the *anaerobes*. There have always been sus-picions that Crohn's is an infection, so it seems reasonable to try this particular medication. It certainly helps some people, but to replace the need for steroids it must be taken in high doses, long term. This may lead to certain side effects that do not manifest in the drug's more familiar usage, to treat vaginal thrush.

Side Effects

- nausea, vomiting
- metallic taste in the mouth
- blackish, furred tongue
- pins and needles
- urticaria (nettle rash)

Very large doses, more than 800 mg daily, for a long period, can lead to a reduction in the number of white cells in the blood (leukope-nia)—which reduces the resistance to infection—also to epileptic fits, and possibly an increased risk of cancer or of harm to an unborn baby. It is wise to take extra care with metronidazole if you are preg-nant, breastfeeding, elderly, or have had liver problems.

Interactions may occur with alcohol, lithium, some antiepilep-tic drugs, and anticlotting medicines.

Although there are many possible side effects, metronidazole is often useful and usually harmless. It is more effective than clo-trimazole or sulfasalazine in controlling the symptoms of Crohn's disease.

IMMUNOSUPPRESSIVES

In 1962 a Dr. Bean introduced 6-mercaptopurine into the treat-ment of both Crohn's disease and ulcerative colitis, following the theory that since some autoimmune disorders occur with Crohn's (see pages 57 and 168), suppressing the immune reactions might have a beneficial effect on the disease itself. Dr. Bean found his drug "little short of miraculous," but then he disappeared into further research. In 1965 nitrogen mustard was tried out—effective, but very toxic.

Azathioprine

Azathioprine, a close relative of Dr. Bean's drug, was brought into use in Crohn's in 1966—with success. In 50 percent of cases it can replace steroids entirely, and it allows a substantial reduction in steroid use in 23 percent.

Side Effects: Azathioprine is very slow in building up an effect. Patients have to try it for four to six months to find out if it is the drug for them.

The danger period for one important side effect is the first three weeks of starting the medicine, when, in the occasional person, it suppresses the blood-making factory in the bone marrow: a serious situation.

Other side effects:

- severe nausea, fever, jaundice

- severe abdominal pain, sometimes with pancreatitis

- diarrhea, which may be mistaken for a relapse of the original illness

Despite this unpleasant list, azathioprine is less toxic than steroids, and some patients have been taking it for as long as 18 years without side effects. It certainly merits a trial when Crohn's is complicated, extensive, or resistant to steroids and other treatments.

Cyclosporine

Cyclosporine came into use for Crohn's in 1984. It is not absorbed in the small intestine in Crohn's sufferers, so it must be administered through a vein. It can be used in those who cannot tolerate or are resistant to steroids.

Side effects: These include a hot feeling in the skin, nausea and vomiting, tremor, overgrowth of the gums, and a tendency for the blood pressure to rise. Cyclosporine interacts with anti-inflammatories in common use.

Methotrexate

Methotrexate (Rheumatrex) is effective in two-thirds of people with Crohn's, but it is toxic. It is used only in those who are chronically ill steroid failures, and those for whom azathioprine has also failed.

Side Effects: These include hair loss, infertility, a lung disorder called pneumonitis, upset to the digestive system, and a low white-cell count.

Interferon

Interferon is sometimes helpful in Crohn's and other chronic disorders. It is administered through an installation tube placed in the colon.

These last few drugs are used in Crohn's when the doctors are scraping the barrel. At such times the surgical option needs serious consideration.

INFLIXIMAB (REMICADE)

The FDA in 1998 approved this new drug for moderate to severe Crohn's disease that does not respond to standard therapies. It is the first treatment approved specifically for Crohn's and the first product documented to reduce the number of open fistulas.

Infliximab is administered intravenously about every eight weeks. It works by blocking the activity of tumor necrosis factor (TNF). TNF is a protein produced by the immune system that may cause the inflammation associated with Crohn's disease. Anti-TNF substances, such as infliximab, remove TNF from the bloodstream before it reaches the intestinal wall, thereby preventing inflammation.

Since infliximab is a new product, tests to ascertain its long-term safety are still being conducted, and only one study has been performed to test its effectiveness in treating Crohn's over the course of several months. This study showed that 62 percent of patients treated with infliximab maintained a clinical response to treatment after 44 weeks (compared with 37 percent of people taking a placebo). However, in people taking azathioprine/6-mercaptopurine concurrently with infliximab, 75 percent showed a clinical response at 44 weeks.

Side Effects

In the study mentioned above, nearly all the patients in the infliximab group as well as in the placebo group reported adverse effects, including upper respiratory tract infection, headache, abdominal pain, nausea, fever, bronchitis, and sore throat. Seven patients (out of a total of 37 taking infliximab) developed human antichimeric antibodies (HACA), an immune response that develops in some people following infliximab treatment due to the drug's combination of human and mouse components.

FISH OIL

Fats or oils are essential for normal life and growth. Fish oils are particularly rich in Omega-3, a type of polyunsaturated fat often lacking in the Western diet. Omega-3 is even better than other polyunsaturates such as sunflower seed oil in protecting against high blood pressure and coronary disease. It is also an excellent anti-inflammatory, and worth a try in Crohn's. Fish oil comes in capsule or liquid form and can be found at natural-foods stores that also sell dietary supplements.

DRUGS STILL UNDERGOING TRIALS

These include the antileprosy drug rifabutin and two antimycobacterial antibiotics, azithromycin and clarithromycin. They all have numerous, unpleasant side effects, and until their efficacy is established, as well as their safety, they are not generally available (see chapter 15). The same precautions apply to thalidomide, the drug so notorious for causing birth defects in infants whose mothers used it during pregnancy. Studies documented late in 1999 showed that thalidomide, traditionally prescribed as a sedative, may be useful in treating patients with severe Crohn's disease who have failed to respond to other therapies. One researcher called the results "dramatic," but everyone involved in the tests emphasized the need for caution—especially with women patients in their childbearing years—and for a large, placebo-controlled study.

Bernard

Bernard was unlucky. He was 45 when he developed Crohn's, well past the regular age of risk, and then he had the unusual misfortune to be resistant to steroids. His main problem was diarrhea. It interfered with every part of his life, but most particularly at work, where he had to keep leaving his desk. Besides, he was losing weight steadily and he felt weak. This was made worse by the anemia: he was passing small amounts of blood on a regular basis, and his ileum was probably unable to absorb the iron he needed. Bernard had the common ileocolonic type of Crohn's, in which both the small and large intestines are involved.

It was disheartening to find that Bernard did not respond to the steroids, but as his doctor said, that still left plenty of choices. Bernard wanted mostly to avoid surgery. He was not eager to take sulfasalazine because of possible damage to his fertility, so his doctor prescribed mesalamine (Pentasa). His symptoms began to settle down, but new ones appeared: he noticed big bruises on his legs when he could not recall any injury; then he had a sore throat. He mentioned it to his doctor, and a blood test showed dyscrasia with a low white-cell count, so the medicine had to be stopped immediately.

Metronidazole, the next option, did nothing for Bernard's diarrhea, but the doctor told him that azathioprine (Imuran), a more powerful drug, would be sure to solve his problems. He should expect to take it for two or three months before they could judge the effect. After enduring for several months a constant feeling of nausea and a horrible metallic taste in his mouth, Bernard was thankful to give up this medicine, too.

Currently he is taking methotrexate (Rheumatrex), and apart from losing most of his hair he has experienced only beneficial effects. The diarrhea is down to three times a day, and Bernard hopes to come off all drugs in a few weeks.

Chapter 9

Treatment Options: Surgery

I t is still something of a mystery how most medicines work, especially in Crohn's disease. There is nothing to see, whereas surgery brings about instant results. Surgeons for the most part have a straightforward approach. Their instinct is to cut out what is diseased and repair what is broken. The ongoing uncertainty about the root cause of Crohn's is frustrating for them, but there are situations in the illness that call for a surgical rescue package.

EMERGENCIES

The chances are a hundred to one against your needing emergency surgery, but like a seatbelt it is good to know it is there for you in a crisis. Emergencies occur when one of the rarer complications of Crohn's arises.

Perforation

This occurs when an ulcer or a fissure extends deeper and deeper into the wall of the intestine until it finally breaks right through, usually into the peritoneal cavity, the inside of the abdomen. There lie the closely packed organs, including stomach, intestines, bladder, and possibly the uterus. Perforation can affect either the small or large intestine, wherever there is a patch of Crohn's. Either way, it is a life-threatening situation, with peritonitis a practical certainty and septicemia a grave threat.

The urgent surgical task is to stop the contents of the gut spilling out, cut away the affected section, and temporarily divert the normal flow of partly processed food away from that section.

Bleeding

Massive bleeding from an ulcerated area occurs most often in the large intestine, but it may have been made worse by a shortage of vitamin K, which is absorbed through the ileum—unless the ileum is affected by Crohn's. Vitamin K is necessary for the blood to clot. Besides our obtaining it from our food, ordinarily it is also manufactured in the large intestine by friendly bacteria. In Crohn's the bacteria are likely to be different, so this backup production of vitamin K may not be available.

A major operation is required to remove the section of intestine, usually in the colon, that is susceptible to hemorrhage. A transfusion of plasma and a concentrate of blood platelets before the operation ensures that clotting can now take place safely. Ideally an angiogram—a map of the arteries in the area—is done before the operation, but this may not be feasible, and time is of the essence. Bleeding from the small intestine calls for resection of the segment involved, but if the colon is affected, total or near-total removal is the best option, with the provision of an ileostomy for waste disposal.

Treatment is essential for the anemia that inevitably results from heavy blood loss (see page 56). Leafy green vegetables supply vitamin K normally, and meat, whole-grain cereals, and legumes provide iron. These are worth prioritizing in the diet for the long term.

Toxic Megacolon

Toxic megacolon occurs in 20 percent of people with Crohn's. It comprises the top emergency in sufferers and is a complication of toxic colitis, a serious condition in itself. An already extensively damaged colon becomes paralyzed and swells up to enormous size, as much as 6 inches across or more. There is imminent danger of perforation, massive hemorrhage, abscess, or septicemia. In this situation *subtotal colectomy* (removal of most of the colon) is the safest treatment, and the sooner the better.

Treatment with medicines, even if it holds the line temporarily, carries a more than 90 percent risk of surgery being needed urgently, often under worse circumstances than if it had been done right away. Nowadays surgeons treat the healthy parts of the bowel very gently, in case they may become of use, and only remove the irrecoverably damaged parts. Antibiotics are used both before the operation and afterwards.

Cancer

Cancer is a complication of very longstanding (ten years or more) disease of the small or large intestine. Cancer of the ileum tends to affect comparatively young men, but more often cancer involves the colon in older people of either sex. Regular checkups, say twice a year, will catch the problem early. They must be thorough and involve viewing (endoscopy) and testing (biopsy).

If a malignant tumor is found, prompt removal is the obvious course, probably with chemotherapy to follow. The outlook for cancer of the colon is particularly hopeful, much better than for other types.

Natalie

Natalie was 21 when she developed toxic megacolon. She had been in remission from Crohn's for several months and liked to tell herself that she had never really had the disease. She certainly did not tell Ned, her new boyfriend, about it. She was on the pill and smoked about 20 cigarettes a day. She drank moderately and liked to boast that she went out every night. Actually, she had been feeling quite ill for a week or two when the acute, unremitting pain gripped her abdomen. It doubled her over and she went into shock. Her roommate found her deadly pale and sweating. The doctor took one look at her, felt her rigidly hard abdominal muscles, and dialed 911. He also rang the hospital. When Natalie arrived the preparations for surgery were already underway. She was given an injection of a wide-spectrum antibiotic almost immediately— no point in wasting time on a culture.

The incision for the operation, which later turned into a scar, went straight down the midline of Natalie's abdomen, to allow easy access to all areas. The diseased colon was removed and a new opening made, bringing the end of the ileum to the surface, an end-ileostomy (see chapter 10). Natalie was woozy for 24 hours after the operation, but able to operate her PCA (patient controlled analgesic) pump. She said she felt weak but was better overall straightaway and made a rapid recovery. She was no longer being poisoned by the toxic colon, the bacteria in the surrounding areas were on the way to being wiped out, and a transfusion had replenished her depleted blood. In fact, Natalie's main complaint was about the thick, hot, constricting antithrombosis stockings that encased her legs.

The ileostomy nurse, who had not had a chance to talk with Natalie before the operation, gave her a crash course in care of the stoma (the incision in her abdomen left by the surgery), and alleviated some of her horror and fear. All Natalie's many friends, especially Ned, rallied around, and at times she was exhausted by their visits and phone calls. But she felt it was worth the effort to be sociable. Natalie has major adjustments to make in her life, but nothing, she says, that she cannot handle.

ELECTIVE SURGERY

Emergency surgery is forced upon you, as though a gun was held to your head. All other surgery is elective, and whether or not you undergo a particular operation, and exactly when, is up to you and your doctor. There is always an alternative, but this is meaningless unless you have some idea of what the choices are. The basic options are laid out below.

Likely reasons for electing surgery include:

- Intractable symptoms—they simply will not get better despite the best medical treatments.

- Chronic obstruction due to a stricture—a narrow stretch in the intestine.

- Fistula—a passageway ulcerated through from the ileum or colon, into:
  - another piece of gut: *enteroenteric, enterocolic.*
  - the vagina: *enterovaginal.*
  - the bladder: *enterovesical.*

- Abscess—a collection of pus, usually connected with a fistula.

- Chronic anemia, from bleeding.

- In children, a failure to thrive, i.e., to grow properly and develop sexually.

Preoperative Preparation

State of Nutrition: This is always important in Crohn's, and vitally so before an operation. The success of surgery depends on being properly nourished beforehand. If necessary, as a boost to your nutrition and to give your intestines a rest, you may have a short period of *parenteral feeding.* A liquid is dripped into a large central vein—usually the subclavian, just under the collarbone—like a blood transfusion, but containing all the nutrients your body needs. Such a "rest period" for the digestive system used to be considered a treatment for Crohn's in itself, but it does not have a lasting effect, and it is too miserable to keep up for long. Two weeks on an elemental diet is another way of augmenting your strength (see chapter 11).

Anemia: Even for those who have been aware of having Crohn's for only a few months, chances are they are anemic. This needs correcting, and the patient will require iron tablets, folate tablets, and B12 injections (see pages 11, 36, 56, 140, 141, 143).

Bowel Preparation: The intestines are washed out (a procedure called *lavage*) the day before the operation. If there is obstruction, or the patient cannot tolerate the lavage procedure, an enema is administered for two days running instead, accompanied by antibiotics.

Antibiotics: Unless there is evidence of sepsis or an abscess, antibiotics by mouth are sufficient. Otherwise they may be included in an enema or injected into a vein. Metronidazole and neomycin are used in most cases.

OPERATIONS FOR CROHN'S DISEASE IN PARTICULAR SITES

Stomach and Duodenum

A peptic ulcer may also be present to confuse the issue, but the usual way Crohn's in this area comes to notice is because of an obstruction caused by the thickened, inflamed lining membranes. The result is intractable vomiting. If the obstruction is in the exit area of the stomach and duodenum, the neatest solution is a *gastrojejunostomy*. The healthy part of the stomach is joined to the jejunum, the section of the small intestine that continues from the duodenum, thus bypassing the blockage.

If only the duodenum is affected, and the stomach lining is healthy, it may be possible to do a *stricturoplasty*, a kind of plastic surgery of the intestine that makes it wider, relieving the tight place without losing any tissue. This is well worthwhile, since with Crohn's of the duodenum, the ileum is almost invariably involved, too, and the less healthy mucous lining you lose from the digestive system the better in the long term. In rare cases with Crohn's the whole stomach may be so unhealthy that it is a relief to have a *gastrectomy*, removal of the stomach itself. This is not as bad as you might suppose, since so much of the digestion is done elsewhere, and a part of the intestine soon stretches to take the place of the stomach. Nevertheless, you need a specially constructed diet and digestive supplements.

Small Intestine

This is the area most typically involved in Crohn's, particularly the ileum. The usual operation is *ileal resection*, cutting out the diseased segments of ileum, often involving 10 to 12 inches of intestine, with resection of the caecum also. Some surgeons prefer a bypass procedure, which preserves more tissue. The drawback here is that it leaves the diseased tissue to molder, outside the mainstream of the alimentary tract. It is then slightly more likely to develop a cancer. The principle of trying to preserve all healthy tissue applies with either method. Once the area with active disease is gone, you are likely to shake off feelings of lethargy, low spirits, and malaise.

Fistulas

In these unwanted passages from one organ to another, so characteristic of Crohn's, there is usually the "villain" piece, the diseased segment of intestine where the ulceration originated, and the "victim" area, which is healthy except where the fistula comes through. This often occurs when Crohn's in the ileum is the source of a fistula into the healthy colon. In this situation only the fistula exit site need be cut out of the colon, plus the track of tissue through which the fistula passes and the diseased segment of ileum.

Fistulas in Particular Areas

Ileosigmoid Fistula: Nine times out of ten this condition starts in the ileum and emerges in the lower (sigmoid) part of the colon. Resection of the diseased part of the ileum is needed, but if the colon looks generally healthy only a small part around the fistula need be removed. The colon can be examined with a sigmoidoscope.

Rectovaginal Fistula: This type of fistula consists of an ulcerated passageway from Crohn's of the rectum tracking through to the vagina. The damaged parts need repairing and the stools temporarily diverted to allow healing to take place. The normal continuity of the colon is restored later.

Colovesical Fistula: These run from colon to bladder, usually showing up through bladder infections and *pneumaturia*—gas or air in the urine (see Edmund, page 62). Removal of the section of colon from which the fistula arose and simple repair of the bladder corrects the problem. While the bladder is healing, a catheter must remain in place for seven to ten days.

Fiona

Fiona had coped with Crohn's disease for five years, since age 27. She was a methodical, rather fastidious person and enjoyed a healthy lifestyle with regular sessions at the gym and the pool, sensible eating, and no cigarettes or alcohol. The only medication she took was an occasional paracetamol for stomachache, and codeine if her bowels were a little loose. It seemed most unfair that someone so careful and meticulous should get this unpleasant-smelling vaginal discharge and horrible pain when she passed a bowel movement.

Even passing a finger as gently as possibly into her anal passage or vagina was painful, so Fiona was given an injection of midazolam to take the edge off the sensations when an endosonograph (an echo picture) was done. The course and position of a fistula from gut to vagina were examined and carefully mapped out to help the surgeon. Medical treatment with metronidazole and another antibiotic, a short course of steroids, and a trial of azathioprine had all failed, so it was a matter of facing the situation. Fiona knew she had Crohn's of the small intestine, but the source of the present trouble was in the rectum. She had to face removal of the rectum and the setting up of a colostomy.

The vagina healed well, and Fiona's dream of having a family remained perfectly possible. She mastered the management of her stoma and acquired a degree of control over its functioning—but her sexual confidence had hit bottom. So she underwent several months of psychotherapy, which rebuilt her self-esteem, and her partner responded to her new, positive attitude. Intercourse is now enjoyable again, and Fiona is hopeful of conceiving. Her newfound self-assurance helps at her job, too.

Stricturoplasty

When there are skip areas scattered along the mucosal lining of the small intestine, a situation characteristic of Crohn's disease, the digestive and absorptive processes are upset. Carbohydrates are not taken in properly, peptic ulcers develop, vitamin B12 is poorly taken up, and the colon is irritated by the arrival of inadequately digested fats and reacts with diarrhea. A low-fat, high-protein diet with no dairy products may help, with supplements of vitamin D and calcium as well as injections of B12. Simple antidiarrheal medicines, such as Imodium (loperamide) or Lomotil (Diphenoxylate) slow the transit time of the material in the gut, allowing a longer period for digestion and absorption. Nevertheless, these maneuvers have only a minimal effect, and weight loss is likely to continue.

More-drastic action is needed, but resection of a long stretch of intestine—to include several separated areas of inflammation—would leave too little of the intestine to perform its vital work of enabling the body to make use of food. This is where the modern operation of stricturoplasty comes in. It relieves the narrowing of the intestine, with its constant propensity to obstruct, without any loss of valuable, irreplaceable tissue. Several stricturoplasties can be done in the same session, which is useful when there are a large number of short strictures separated by healthy intestine, or when several segments of the ileum have already been resected and there are no more that can be spared.

The operation is simple. A longitudinal incision is made over the narrow part of the gut, but it is sewn up horizontally, widening its shape. Complications are rare after stricturoplasty.

In extensive disease, a combination of stricturoplasty, as much as possible, and resection, as little as possible, may be the best solution.

Crohn's Colitis

Although Dr. Crohn said it could not happen, it is no rarity for the colon alone to be affected by Crohn's disease. Such a condition, called Crohn's colitis, can be recognized by features similar to those in disease of the small intestine—a variety of different types of ulcer, from superficial to very deep, skip areas, fistulas, and involvement of the full thickness of the gut wall.

Crohn's colitis is more common in males of all ages and seniors of either sex. There are three surgical possibilities:

- If an isolated patch of Crohn's is the only sign of disease in the colon, it is worth trying resection of that part only. It leaves the patient with a chance of normal bowel function, including passing bowel movements normally, for several years. Further surgery is usually necessary in the long term.

- If several segments are diseased, those parts only are removed, leaving the rectum and anus to work in the ordinary way (a procedure called subtotal colectomy).

- Resection of the whole colon, including the last part of the alimentary system (proctocolectomy), often becomes necessary in the end. An ileostomy is constructed.

The first operation listed above depends on the rectum and anus being virtually free of disease. In this case there is a 30 percent chance of the desired outcome, with no need of further major treatment. In 35 percent of patients, the symptoms return after the operation, and the remaining lower part of the colon has to be resected and a colostomy or ileostomy made. Some people are so anxious to avoid this that they refuse the operation and struggle on with medicines, even when their symptoms are increasingly troublesome.

The big nuisance about Crohn's disease is that even if you have surgery, it is not likely to be the end of the matter. Crohn's can start up again anywhere. The recurrence rate of symptoms after all but one of the operations for Crohn's runs at about 50 percent—but, on the other hand, you also have great powers of recovery. Proctocolectomy, removal of the whole large bowel including the anus and rectum, involves a risk of relapse of only 10 to 25 percent.

Ano-rectal Crohn's Disease

In this type, typically, deep fissures, fistulas, or an abscess appear in the ano-rectal area, and passing a stool can be agonizingly painful. Suppositories help in mild cases, but surgery is usually needed. Surgery can relieve any constriction in the anus, while dilators may be useful to prevent its narrowing down again. Metronidazole (Flagyl) is definitely beneficial in Crohn's of this area and makes the surgery safer, but it is an adjunct, not a substitute for the operation. There is little evidence of metronidazole benefiting Crohn's in the ileum or upper colon.

Any child or teenager with unusual symptoms or appearances in the anal area needs a full diagnostic investigation to eliminate the possibility of sexual abuse.

Crohn's Disease of the Appendix

Crohn's of the appendix only is a real rarity. The treatment is a standard appendectomy. More often the symptoms will suggest acute appendicitis, and while the appendix may or may not be healthy, inflammation is seen at the lower end of the ileum: *terminal ileitis*. If the colon is also involved the condition is called *ileocolitis*. Most surgeons remove only the appendix if the tissues immediately surrounding it look healthy, but leave the appendix if there is a risk of making the Crohn's inflammation worse, and start medical treatment. In the rare situations where Crohn's of the end part of the ileum—the caecum—and the appendix is causing obstruction, or the inflammation near the appendix is so severe that the tissues are breaking down, the only course is to cut out all the diseased area and make an ileostomy.

RELAPSE AND RECURRENCE

Most patients will need surgery at some stage in the course of their Crohn's, and there is an unlucky group who relapse regularly so that they have to undergo repeated operations. They eventually take the surgery in stride, and malnutrition becomes the major problem. It is because of these people that the concept of minimal removal of tissue has caught on, replacing the old idea of taking it all away in the vain hope of getting rid of the disease. The game plan that evolved in the 1990s was to remove as little as possible. It has been shown that once Crohn's has been diagnosed it can appear spontaneously anywhere in the alimentary system, without direct spread from a diseased area.

Another disappointing factor is that no medicine has been found so far that reliably prevents recurrence. As with everything in Crohn's, there is a variety of different views and ideas. The good news is that the large pharmaceutical companies and surgical research departments are working nonstop following leads to improve the situation.

TOXIC COLITIS

Toxic colitis can be either the first intimation of Crohn's disease or a development in the course of a long illness. It is more serious than the more common Crohn's colitis, with the constant threat of a lethal complication, toxic megacolon. Even without the danger-ous enlargement of the colon, surgery is regarded as urgent in most cases. The deciding factors are:

- Diarrhea: more than six bowel movements daily.

- Weight loss of more than 10 percent.

- Abdominal pain.

- Pulse higher than 100 beats per minute.

- Temperature higher than 102.3°F.

- Distended abdomen.

- Colon appearing enlarged in X-ray.

- Laboratory tests showing a high white-cell count and low albumin (protein) in the blood.

Increasing abdominal distension, indicating the development of megacolon, is the signal for immediate action. The operation must be radical, involving one of the following:

- Proctocolectomy—resection of the whole colon to the anus, plus an end-ileostomy.

- Subtotal colectomy and end-ileostomy—by far the most frequent operation, and healing is usually trouble-free.

These used to be dangerous procedures, but these days the situation has changed dramatically for the better. This is partly because doctors are more likely to make the diagnosis earlier and start treatment, including surgery, sooner, and also because the dangers of toxic megacolon are widely recognized and looked for. In addition, sufferers today are more willing to accept surgery as inevitable. Better antibiotics and more sophisticated aftercare mean that convalescence is shorter and patients are less liable to suffer setbacks. You can concentrate on "rebooting" your life, including special care for your nourishment.

Richard

Richard was 33. As long as he could remember, he had been perfectly fit until out of the blue he began having nonstop abdominal pain, with eight or nine bowel movements a day. He felt dehydrated but vomited if he drank anything, and his temperature hovered around 105°F. Weight had fallen off him like he had taken off an overcoat, but he felt unaccountably happy and important. His doctor found that his heart was pounding away at 150 beats a minute. The clear advice was that he should undergo urgent surgery, but Richard was adamant that he would rather die than live with an ileostomy.

He was put on huge doses of steroids, antidiarrheals, antibiotics, and immunosuppressives—but with no appreciable improvement. In fact, a new sinister symptom showed up—Richard's abdomen began to swell, and his euphoria turned to delirium. It was only then, when his judgement was obviously impaired and his parents—his next of kin—gave their permission for surgery, that Richard had the operation that saved his life. He had the standard subtotal colectomy and ileostomy, and his steroid dosage was gradually reduced.

It took Richard several months to recover fully, mentally as well as physically, but he did learn to cope with his stoma and get back to his career in computers and the rock band that filled his leisure time.

Chapters 8 and 9 have provided information about the basic medical and surgical treatments available in Crohn's. They may seem daunting, but the wide areas of lifestyle, attitude, diet, and personal psychology are equally important. In these areas you, the patient, have much more choice and control.

A mass of evidence suggests that whatever else applies—infection, autoimmunity or other immunity problems, genetics—one's environment has a major influence on the progress of the illness. Why is Crohn's so common in temperate climates such as North America and Northern Europe compared with hot, sunny Africa and Southern Europe? How do smoking, the contraceptive pill, sugar, and stress fit in? There is still much to be discovered. Meanwhile, you have many positive options for keeping yourself well while in remission and to help matters during an attack.

Chapter 10

Ileostomy and Colostomy

rohn's patients find it hard when they are told they must undergo a surgical procedure that means they will have to pass their bowel movements through an artificial opening in the front of the abdomen, instead of going to the bathroom in the ordinary way. Such an operation is either an ileostomy, which connects to the small intestine, or a colostomy, connecting to the colon. In either case the new exit is called a *stoma* (Greek for mouth). In the case of a colostomy the stoma is usually made below and to the left of the navel, while an ileostomy stoma is placed low down on the right.

A patient requiring such a procedure may feel that having a stoma is the end of the world, that she or he will be different from everybody else. In fact, he or she is joining a club with more than a million members in the United States, with another 15,000 joining every year. The reason these figures seem high is that some colostomies, in particular, are temporary. You won't know who the other club members are unless you are close friends, but they can be anywhere: working in offices, selling in shops, practicing any profession, swimming in the local pool.

Of course, you may still feel that you would prefer anything to having the operation—until you consider the alternative. Often a colostomy or ileostomy saves your life, and in all cases it will relieve a great deal of suffering.

REASONS FOR HAVING AN ILEOSTOMY OR COLOSTOMY

Emergency Situations

Perforation: When the Crohn's ulcerates right through the gut wall, spilling its contents into the abdomen, it will lead to fatal peritonitis without immediate surgery.

Intestinal Obstruction: This is another life-or-death situation. The first case record of a successful colostomy was in 1792. A baby was born without an anus—congenital obstruction. Death seemed inevitable until, on the third day, the desperate measure of making an opening into the colon was performed. The baby lived. If a narrowing or stricture of the small intestine becomes completely blocked so that nothing can pass down the alimentary canal, it is urgent to provide another escape route for the waste. Nearly all those with classic Crohn's disease will need surgery sooner or later, because strictures are so common.

Massive Hemorrhage from the Colon: Heavy bleeding is not unusual in Crohn's affecting the colon—Crohn's colitis—and if you have lost four units or more of blood you need urgent surgery to prevent further loss.

Toxic Colitis: This is a dangerous development in Crohn's colitis and requires prompt action.

Toxic Megacolon: This is the top emergency—toxic megacolon is a colon that has become huge and paralyzed.

There is no question of delay in any of these conditions, but in others there may be time to discuss and prepare beforehand.

Nonemergency Reasons for Ostomy Surgery

While some situations do not call for immediate action, an operation may still be necessary:

- To avoid unpleasant or hazardous complications, for example, bowel cancer. Long-standing Crohn's, especially if it has lasted ten years or more, increases the risk of small-intestine cancer six-fold compared with the norm, and nearly as much for colon cancer. Young men are the most susceptible to small-intestine cancer and older people of both sexes to colon cancer. It is foolhardy to struggle on indefinitely with a cocktail of medications that fails to control the illness satisfactorily.

- To put an end to chronic partial obstruction that is causing increasingly frequent colicky abdominal pain, with the ever present threat of complete blockage.

- Continuing failure to grow in children and adolescents: if nothing is done they will remain stunted and poorly equipped sexually.

- Long-standing generally poor health, so that you hardly ever feel totally well—despite trying all the medicines, diets, and alternative therapies.

- Physical complications such as fistula or abscess.

- Chronic anemia, caused by persistent, though slight, bleeding from the anal passage. The symptoms may include fatigue and shortness of breath (see pages 36 and 56–58).

Patients need have no fear that a knife-happy surgeon will persuade them into an operation they don't need or remove more tissue than is absolutely necessary. The key word for surgery in Crohn's is conservatism. Your doctors will preserve as much healthy tissue as possible, and only severely diseased parts of the intestine that can never function usefully again will be resected (cut out). Of course, patients will have the major hurdles of getting over the operation and of adjusting to new toilet arrangements, but the end result is that they will feel fitter than they have for ages. With the removal of the diseased tissue, many of its ill effects, both obvious and more subtle, are taken away too.

Ellie

Ellie had a difficult childhood. Her elderly father died when she was five, and her mother dated a series of male friends who turned out to be no good. The last one tried to seduce Ellie, who was then only 14, and it was in the following year that Ellie developed ano-rectal Crohn's disease. She experienced continual rectal discomfort, diarrhea on and off, and pain when passing a stool. Treatment with metronidazole, other antibiotics and various steroid ointments helped briefly, but the illness kept getting worse.

A colostomy provided considerable relief. Ano-rectal Crohn's never goes into satisfactory, long-term remission with only drug treatment. Without the disabling symptoms and reliance on a constantly changing regimen of ineffective medication, Ellie was able to live a near-normal teenage life. Music was the catalyst that enabled her to make friends on equal terms with her own generation. That was eight years ago. Now she is engaged to marry a violinist in a well-known orchestra. Something is going right for her.

BEFORE THE OPERATION

Except in the severest emergencies, your surgeon will want to know as much as possible about the state of affairs inside your abdomen before she or he operates. The test procedures (already explained in chapter 7) are nothing to worry about and may include:

- Barium enema—a liquid containing barium, which shows up on an X-ray, is administered like an ordinary enema. It outlines the inside of the colon. The procedure is vaguely uncomfortable but not painful, and it takes less than half an hour.

- Ultrasound—not unpleasant at all, but you have to drink a lot of water beforehand so that your bladder lifts the other parts into the best position for viewing.

- CT (computerized tomography) scan—a comprehensive type of X-ray.

- Sigmoidoscopy—a flexible tube with a light at the end is

passed into the anal passage so that the operator has a direct view of the inside of the storage colon. The procedure takes 20 to 30 minutes but is no worse than uncomfortable.

- Colonoscopy—a fiber-optic instrument provides a view of the whole of the lining of the large intestine, and enables tissue samples to be taken (biopsy) to examine under the microscope. You will be given a mild sedative during the colonoscopy, which takes about 30 minutes. It is the best available test and provides the best and most detailed information.

- Ileocolonoscopy—a colonoscopy which includes the ileum.

AFTER THE OPERATION

You will have already met your stoma-care nurse before the operation. Now you will be partners in getting to know your stoma and how best to keep it happy and functioning well. You will not be left to struggle on your own with this new, strange arrangement. Although it may be hard to believe, you *will* get used to it. It takes about three weeks to learn the essentials, three months to become expert enough to feel confident, and the rest of the year to complete your emotional adjustment.

Whether you have had an ileostomy or a colostomy, the essential equipment is a bag to collect the waste matter. With a colostomy the waste is like a soft stool. The material from an ileostomy, which has been less completely processed in the digestive system, is semiliquid, like rather runny porridge. It is not possible to control the elimination process after an ileostomy, but with a colostomy, you can acquire a useful degree of control over its action in three or four months. The equipment in either case may be one piece or two pieces: either simply a disposable bag that fits over the stoma, or a base plate over the stoma to which the disposable bag is clipped. Ileostomy bags may have a drain, so that you can empty them without removing them. For sports or some other activities you may want to empty the bag before it is completely full.

The new toilet regime takes more time and more care than the old way, but soon becomes part of your daily routine. Diabetics are in a similar situation, but they have even more complex and fussy health rituals—and strict dietary constraints to boot. The many elderly people with incontinence problems also learn to cope with various appliances, and even the healthiest young women have menstrual periods to deal with.

COMING TO TERMS AND LIVING A FULL LIFE

It takes character and persistence to win out against Crohn's, even with the support of loved ones and professional help and encouragement. Your emotions take a hard knock, and you are bound to feel both anxious and depressed at first.

Anxiety

Anxiety, sometimes approaching panic, is natural and normal when you face the new situation of having a stoma. Leakage is a big fear, and the ultimate horror is that the bag will come unattached, leaving a terrible mess. This is extremely unlikely, though, because the appliances are made to fit well and the waterproof adhesive is extremely strong. Nevertheless, it is a good idea always to carry with you a set of spares, including underwear and a sponge bag; this is your insurance policy. Then all you need to set things right until you get home is the nearest restroom.

Apart from this disaster scenario, which is not so terrible in any event, there are a number of lesser but more pervasive worries.

- *Other people will notice a smell.* No more likely than with anyone else. The most unpleasant, permeating human odor is that of sweat, especially from smelly feet and unwashed clothes. As you can see, these do not apply to Crohn's-related conditions.

- *The bulge of the bag is very obvious under the clothes.* Not unless you wear a skintight leotard. It is hardly noticeable even with a swimsuit, especially if the fabric is patterned.

- *The stoma is repulsive.* It is normally healthy tissue, and no more unsightly than, for instance, the sexual organs.

- *You cannot enjoy any normal pleasures, so you are cut off from your friends.* Not true. It takes a little more trouble, but you can swim, play sports, dance, and have sex (see below). There is a minipouch to use during periods of physical activity and a sports belt to make things more secure.

If feelings of anxiety are interfering with your life, even when there is no special reason for them, it is worth learning some mind- and muscle-relaxation techniques from a psychologist or an occupational therapist. Ask your physician for a referral. Audiocassettes containing guided visualizations are also available. Breathing-control exercises are useful if you are prone to hyperventilate, and breathing in and out of a paper bag is a handy first-aid maneuver.

Depression

As with anxiety, it would be unnatural if you did not feel a sense of loss and some sadness when you first have a stoma. The operation can come as a blow to your self-esteem—although you may understand logically that you are still the same person and worth just as much. A wide range of negative emotions can grip you. Some people even feel guilty or ashamed—as though they are somehow at fault. Yet, do you blame other people when they have an illness, or think less of them? Of course not. Nor will your friends.

Ordinary acquaintances will not know the situation and will judge you by the usual measures: kindness, cheerfulness, sense of humor—and most important of all, your interest in them. Of course you will experience bouts of frustration and irritation plus a touch of anger of the "why me" variety. You are not going to turn into a saint so don't criticize yourself, and don't try to be perfect.

If you are unable to argue yourself out of negative feelings and you feel low and hopeless most of the time, like life is not worth living, it is time to get help. This may mean talking with a counselor or psychotherapist, but if you are losing sleep and weight you may wish to see a psychiatrist who can give you antidepressant medication as well as, but not instead of, the therapy.

RELATIONSHIPS, INTIMACY, AND SEX

The single most important concern after the operation, when the life-and-death issues are out of the way, is sex. There may not have been time to discuss this in advance, so a man may be uninformed and fearful that he has lost his potency—as 55-year-old William put it, "be only half a man." While men fret about performance, women are afraid that having a stoma will be such a turn-off that no one could ever want them again.

For those who are married or in a stable relationship the fear is that their sex life will be in ruins, their partner can no longer love them, and the marriage will collapse. In the majority of cases sexual habits continue much as before, and the couple remains in the same relationship.

The physical effects of the operation are mild. A man may have a slight fall-off in his ability to maintain an erection, while a woman may find she can no longer achieve multiple orgasms. Much more important is the psychological effect. Sexual success is 90 percent a matter of attitude and confidence. A follow-up of stoma patients in the 1970s found that after the operation:

- 85 percent found intercourse easy, compared with 89 percent before.

- 57 percent had about the same interest in sex, 21 percent had less, and 22 percent more.

- 75 percent of the men could keep their erection satisfactorily, compared with 92 percent before.

- 87 percent of both sexes could achieve orgasm, compared with 90 percent preoperatively.

Not too bad a score, but psychotherapy is essential for those who cannot adjust sexually to the new arrangements. It usually takes about 12 months to recover from the operation and to adjust physically and psychologically. The partner also needs time to adjust, and joint therapy sessions can be useful. On a practical level, preparing for sex means emptying the bag and changing to a mini, or strapping it up out of the way, bathing, and powdering, and covering the stoma area with adapted underwear.

Rita

Rita and Denby had been together for six years and had a three-year-old daughter. Rita had struggled to cope with her Crohn's with fair success until she was 32, when she developed a fistula between the small intestine and the womb. It made her life miserable, and she was advised to undergo a resection of parts of the ileum and colon, with an ileostomy. Her relationship with Denby had often been stormy, and sex was at the core of their problems. Denby found that he was now impotent with Rita—but not with other women. He would not go along with counseling, so Rita, a girl of spirit, said they should separate and found a therapist.

She became increasingly independent, confident—and attractive—and after one short-term affair met a man who really appreciated her, made love to her, and suggested marriage. Rita's little girl and Ed's young son have also benefited from their mutually supportive relationship.

For the so far uncommitted, the problems are different. For ordinary social activities your slogan must be *just do it*—don't chicken out. The tricky part is when you meet someone with whom an intimate relationship is likely and sex a real possibility. The difficult decision is when to tell him or her about the stoma. Obviously, it is not the first thing you talk about with someone new, but it is a good idea to mention, early on, that you have had a major operation, and that it was for Crohn's disease. Crohn's has no unfavorable connotations.

Anyone whose feelings change when you tell them about the stoma is obviously not for you. For all practical purposes it is no worse than having a part of your body under a bandage for some reason. Your sexual feelings are not reduced by the physical change, nor is your fertility. Crohn's disease is no bar to pregnancy, and there are numerous cases of happy and successful mothers who conceived after an ostomy operation.

The key is your emotional reaction. To ensure a successful adjustment, most people need a therapist—since reassurance from someone who knows is a vital ingredient—as well as a sympathetic partner. Ignore anyone who expects you to be satisfied just to be alive. Life is for living *and* enjoying.

EMBARRASSING SITUATIONS

There is no denying that you need some creativity and a sense of humor when you must live with a stoma. You are bound to run into some embarrassing situations.

- Your stomach gurgles loudly—grin and say it is the aftereffect of an operation.

- The bag gets full of gas and bulges, with the risk of making a smell—excuse yourself and release the gas in private.

- You are aware of a leakage. No need for panic; just get to a restroom and bring your emergency pack into play.

- Nosy people try to bring the conversation around to how you cope with a stoma—don't be offended, be brief. Let it be understood that it is no more remarkable than any other private bodily function. No one wants to discuss how they clean their false teeth, either.

EATING AND DRINKING

These can contribute to the embarrassing situations. There are no general dietary do's and don'ts for people with a stoma; it's a matter of finding out what suits you individually. This is a good time to take a preliminary peek at chapters 11 through 13, dealing with diet. There are a number of problems that are likely to crop up in connection with your stoma.

Gas

We all produce a certain amount, from babyhood onwards. Some of it we swallow and some is produced in the gut, from our food. It can be embarrassing when it escapes through the stoma, or worse, gets trapped and causes discomfort and a bulge.

Swallowing air comes from smoking, gulping your food down, talking with your mouth full, putting more food in before it is empty, and drinking and eating at the same time. So—this is the time to give up smoking, if you ever did, to avoid chewing gum, to eat with your mouth shut, and to avoid huge mouthfuls. Chew your food thoroughly, so that it slides down easily. They say a ripe banana, mashed up in your mouth, is very helpful in preventing air-swallowing.

Food and drink that cause gas include fizzy drinks and alcohol; beans, peas, and corn; cabbage, cauliflower, and spinach; mushrooms, turnips, and nuts; and, for some people, milk and milk products.

Unpleasant Smell

This applies to other people's waste, too. Watch out for the effects of asparagus, garlic, baked beans, the cabbage family, eggs, and fish. The ostomy patient is more aware of any smell because with the new arrangement both gas and waste come out in front—right under the nose. As far as other people are concerned, however, your fart is no more noticeable than anybody else's.

Loose or Too Frequent Bowel Movements

These often result from nervous tension. If you are feeling anxious, talk about the feeling and get it ironed out. Culprits on the dietary front are raw fruit, dried fruit, spinach, baked beans, chocolate, and highly spiced dishes.

Constipation

If nothing is turning up in the bag or just a watery fluid that has percolated around harder feces, you need to get your doctor's help and advice. You want to avoid a blockage, and it may be that some medication you are taking has a constipating effect, for example, iron pills or painkillers.

Odd-Colored Stools

This is a not-to-worry phenomenon, unless the color is due to blood. Nine times in ten it is caused by staining from a red food dye; fruits such as strawberries, blackberries, or blueberries; licorice; iron pills; or beets.

Remember that you are not a machine, and your stoma is a part of you that, like other parts, may not always work perfectly. "Growing pains" may crop up in the first few months. Most of them are concerned with your learning the ropes, but the two important problems are obstruction and abscess. Since the stoma is so accessible, treatment is much easier than it would be if the trouble were hidden inside your abdomen.

Ian

Ian, 67, had been a lifelong smoker—a two-pack-a-day man— and he had suffered from Crohn's disease since the age of 45. So far he had gotten by on a cocktail of pills and two localized operations for stricture. He had enjoyed some long periods of remission, but these were getting shorter and his symptoms were troublesome. He was chronically anemic and his weight was on the slide.

A new, enthusiastic young resident at the hospital decided to give Ian and his treatment regimen a complete overhaul, including colonoscopy and biopsy. Under the microscope the sample of tissue from Ian's colon showed *dysplasia*: a change from the normal structure. It was a warning of the likelihood of cancer developing. This did not mean panicking, since on average there is a two- to three-year grace period from the stage of premalignancy to cancer itself. The diseased colon was removed and a colostomy constructed. Ian's wife has been a tower of strength. She is glad to have him alive.

SOME SPECIAL SITUATIONS

Travel

Always have your contingency supplies with you, and in your carry-on bags pack twice as much of the stoma-care materials as you think you need. It is also useful to locate the airport medical facilities as a matter of routine. When Vivienne went to Rome, her baggage flew on to Jerusalem, but she had her emergency supplies to cover the situation until she could get to a doctor and a pharmacy. You may wish to take a plastic sheet with you to protect the hotel bedsheets against any accident, but a towel is a lot more comfortable. Either precaution is more to ease your anxiety than to relieve a genuine problem.

Sports

Your stoma is as tough and resilient as any other healthy tissue. You do not need to feel that it is made of Dresden china. A sports belt to keep the bag in place will add to your sense of security, and for a swimsuit choose a bold pattern so the bulge will not be noticeable. You do not need to worry that water will cause the appliance to come loose. The special adhesive is stronger when it is wet.

Driving

Because your whole abdomen has been through a major procedure you should avoid the twisting and turning movements that arise when you drive until your body has had time to heal. Allow a month after your operation before you get behind the wheel again.

Work

It is essential for your psyche to get back to work as soon as it is sensible to do so. When that will be depends on the type of work you do. Heavy lifting is out for good. Because you have had major surgery, your body will be using its resources for repair and reconstruction. You cannot expect to have the energy, physical or mental, to manage a normal job, however sedentary, for three months. Even then it is wise to start by working part-time—shorter or fewer days. This will enable you to keep in touch with your work and with what is going on in your body.

Your prescription reads: sleep, rest, food, and company. The last two are the most important—nourishment for your body and your mind. As for reading material, a must is Dr. Craig White's book *Positive Options for Living with Your Ostomy* (Hunter House, 2002).

Because of my connection with the gastroenterology department of a hospital and my special interest in a group of brave people tackling the difficulties that can pop up in Crohn's disease, I cannot help knowing which of the people I see in and around the hospital have a stoma. There is that nice man at the library, for one, and the girl at the lingerie counter in the department store; then there is the middle-aged couple who run the newsstand—she is the one with Crohn's—and the bank manager. There must be plenty of others I don't know about, living perfectly normal lives (with whatever effort it takes)—working, playing, laughing, and loving.

Chapter 11

Diet in Prevention
and Treatment

he key to coping successfully with Crohn's disease is how
well one eats. To start with, good nutrition is important to
minimize the risk of developing the illness. Since good
nutrition has been known for decades to be a protection against
infection with Mycobacterium tuberculosis, it is reasonable to
expect this also applies to its cousin, Mycobacterium paratuberculosis. Good nutrition is particularly important for those who have a
family member with either form of IBD, ulcerative colitis or
Crohn's disease.

CONVENIENCE, JUNK, AND FAST FOODS

We know that people who make a habit of eating convenience
foods—the polite term for junk food—stand a bigger chance of
developing Crohn's disease. The special villains are white refined
sugar and white refined flour, our universal Western addictions.
Cookies, cakes, doughnuts, pasta, white bread, and hamburger
buns—all are on the "bad food" list. Yet they are so handy just to
pick up and eat.

Sugar

Most prepackaged convenience foods, including such items as

breakfast cereals, frozen dinners, baked beans, canned soups, packaged lunch meats, and certain processed baby foods are laced with white sugar. The aim is to increase their palatability, since nowadays our tastes have been trained from babyhood to accept sweetness as standard. Natural flavors seem insipid.

Pure, white sugar can be used by your body as fuel for your brain and your muscles, and any surplus is stored as body fat, but it makes no contribution to building and repair work, which is necessary in ordinary health and even more so during an illness. It is standard procedure for your body to renew its various parts in a continuous cycle. For example, your red blood cells are replaced by new ones every six weeks, your skin is renewed every two or three weeks, and the lining of your intestines replaces itself twice a week. Modern refined and processed foods have had the vital nourishment removed from them.

Fats and Oils

The other foods to watch out for are certain kinds of fat, either saturated fats from animal sources, hydrogenated vegetable fats, or polyunsaturated fats that have been heated—for instance cooking with sunflower seed oil. As a nation Americans eat too much fat, especially the saturated type in dairy products and meat, and this contributes to a high level of coronary heart disease and cancer, especially of the colon—which is related to long-term Crohn's disease. For Crohn's patients it is even more important to watch dietary fat intake. The damaged intestines cannot process fats efficiently, and this causes a train of problems. The exception is fish oil.

Additives

Junk food in general, with its artificial colorings, flavorings, and preservatives, increases the risk of Crohn's. The object of most of the additives is to improve the appearance and prolong the shelf life of the product—not to increase its nutritional value. You must have noticed grapefruit and apples from far-flung places looking very attractive with a high polish. They have been waxed, to keep them looking good longer. The downside is that the vitamins will have almost disappeared by the time you get to eat them.

Fancied-up, processed foods, especially the fatty and sugary ones, are best avoided. If you like a cigarette with your meal, try to drop that, too. It interferes with taste. You will find that after a short time you will begin to appreciate the subtler natural flavor of fruits, vegetables, whole grains, and protein foods—eggs, cheese, fish, and meat—that have not been made into prepackaged meals and sausages.

The only other item in general use that is known to make you very slightly more susceptible to Crohn's is the birth-control pill.

FOOD INTOLERANCE

One of the long-established theories about the causes of Crohn's disease is food intolerance, by analogy with *celiac disease*. Certainly some people with Crohn's, but by no means all, find that particular foods make their symptoms worse. The lucky ones find that if they cut out these foods their illness goes into remission.

The food sensitivity or intolerance associated with Crohn's is not an allergy. Allergic reactions are usually obvious and immediate, and the tiniest quantity of the allergen—the substance responsible—is enough to set off the symptoms. Skin-prick testing produces a reaction in allergy, but not in Crohn's food intolerance. With Crohn's a substantial amount of the specific food is required and the response comes on slowly. Since nutrition is of fundamental importance in Crohn's, it is worth exploring seriously which foods are good for you, and especially which you must avoid. There is no virtue in making yourself eat something your body rejects, either through the bowels or with abdominal pain.

You could be one of those whose Crohn's lays low as long as they keep to their personal restrictions. Some foods you would not miss if you never ate them again, but you are more likely to react to something you eat frequently. It is often, though not invariably, the protein in the problem food that causes the trouble.

A long list of foodstuffs known to bring on symptoms in some people is given below. You will not be sensitive to all of them, but it is likely that if a particular food induces your symptoms, it will not be the only one. That is why it often does not work to try and find out if a specific food is the culprit simply by omitting it from your diet for a week or two. Even if you hit on one food that does not agree with you, the chances are that you will still be eating another one just as bad, and your symptoms will continue. To do the detective work effectively you need the determination to spend many weeks on an elimination diet—for which your doctor's supervision is essential. For Crohn's sufferers it is not safe to disrupt an already precarious state of nutrition without expert monitoring.

The foodstuffs that head the list of suspects include wheat, dairy products, the brassica (cabbage) family, corn or maize, yeast, tomatoes, citrus fruit, and eggs.

Milk and Dairy products

One item that crops up frequently in Crohn's is sensitivity to *lactose*, or milk sugar, which is present in all milk products. The basic problem is a genetic shortage of *lactase*, the enzyme that processes this specific sugar so that the milk can be digested and absorbed. Lactase deficiency is not uncommon, but Crohn's can point it up, and symptoms occur in reaction to milk in any form. It is particularly in evidence after an ileostomy. However, it is a mistake to deny yourself such valuable foods as milk, cheese, and yogurt, unless you are sure that doing so makes a substantial difference for the better. The most versatile substitute for cow's milk is made from soy—most brands contain sugar to improve or disguise the taste—but you may be able to take sheep or goat's milk. Several flavors of soy "cheeses" are available, but they often contain small amounts of milk solids to enhance melting. Tofu, Chinese for soybean curd, can also serve as a cheese substitute.

Wheat

In wheat the troublemaker is likely to be gluten. Fortunately there is a range of gluten-free wheat products available in natural-food stores and some supermarkets, but they are expensive. Rye bread, so long as it is 100 percent rye, is not too expensive and can be found in most supermarkets. Oatcakes, rice cakes and crackers, and rye crackers can fill a niche.

Yeast

If yeast is causing the trouble you can switch to soda bread, pita bread, naan (from India), matzos, and other flatbreads (unleavened). The largest quantities of yeast appear in bouillon cubes, beer, wine, cider, and vitamin B tablets. You also need to be careful of pickles, dressings, and cheeses, but liquor is usually tolerated well, in moderation. The United States enjoys strict food-labeling laws, so read the ingredient list on any prepackaged food before purchasing it.

Brassicas

It is easy to avoid the cabbage family and to eat your green vegetables as spinach, lettuce, and green peppers—plus those other vegetables, the legumes.

Tomatoes

Similarly, tomatoes can be avoided but may crop up in disguise in soups, pizzas, and other premade dishes. However, you may find that it is only raw tomatoes that cause trouble and that you are able to eat cooked or canned ones.

Eggs

Look out for *lecithin* among the list of ingredients in manufactured foods. Otherwise, remember the egg in pancakes, waffles, quiches, egg noodles and pasta, cakes and other baked goods, and mayonnaise and other dressings. There is no easy way of substituting for eggs, so if you are a vegetarian, check that you are not depriving yourself of the B vitamins. Other sources include whole grains, green vegetables, nuts, and seeds—and for vitamin B12 you must have some food of animal origin.

Maize, Corn

Besides canned, fresh, or frozen corn, watch out for cornbread, polenta, grits and hominy, cornmeal in soups, custards, gravy powder, and sauces. It is also in cornflakes and some other breakfast cereals—so it was not such a crazy idea when someone suggested cornflakes were the cause of Crohn's disease (see page 20).

The idea of food intolerance as an important cause of Crohn's disease has often been dismissed—with some justification, since obviously it does not apply in all cases. Nevertheless, for some people it is the answer. Might such a condition not make the intestines susceptible to infection, perhaps by upsetting immunity balances? It was Dr. John Hunter of Addenbrooke's Hospital in Cambridge, England, who first took the idea seriously and carried out a series of scientifically planned, clinical trials, using a special, elemental diet.

ELEMENTAL DIETS

These diets contain no food—as we know it—nor microorganisms. They are constructed from ordinary foods that have been broken down into their constituent chemicals, and then into the smallest and simplest molecules. Proteins, for example, are separated into amino acids. The result is a liquid that tastes horrible.

Several elemental diets, available by prescription only in the United States, are manufactured. As well as being extremely unpalatable, they are expensive, but if you have been diagnosed with Crohn's your insurance may cover them. Because of the taste, half the people who try drinking an elemental diet soon give up, so the standard way of taking it is through the nose! A soft, flexible tube is slipped into one nostril, down the back of the throat and into the stomach or duodenum. This way you do not smell it and it bypasses the taste buds. The tube does not feel as unpleasant as you might think. I found I barely noticed it after a few minutes, and you do not have to be in the hospital to pour down measured doses of the "diet" at the appropriate times.

The elemental diet is used in two ways: as the first stage in an elimination procedure, or as a treatment in itself. Either way, the point is that while you are taking this liquid you are not having any food that could trigger an attack or relapse of Crohn's. The absence of whole proteins is especially important.

Reasons for Using an Elemental Diet

* as one option in case of an acute attack
* as an adjunct to steroid treatment when progress is unsatisfactory
* undernutrition
* as a build-up before an operation
* pregnancy
* failure to grow in a child or adolescent
* the patient is a young child

An elemental diet sounds dull and bleak, but it is nutritious. Delivered straight into the duodenum, it is full of calories ready to be absorbed.

Results After Two to Four Weeks on the Diet

* Remission of symptoms in 80 to 90 percent of acute cases.
* Weight gain, particularly in Crohn's of the small intestine only, fairly effective if both large and small bowels are involved, but less so if only the colon is affected. Similarly, relapse is less likely after the diet if it is the upper reaches of the gut that are affected.
* Increased albumin in the blood, showing that protein loss is being corrected.
* Hemoglobin level rises, showing correction of anemia.
* ESR lower, showing a reduction in inflammation.
* Intestinal permeability reduced.

Intestinal permeability: If the gut lining is damaged by Crohn's disease, this allows bacteria to work their way deeply into the intestinal wall, causing deep ulcers, fissures, and fistulas. One theory about Crohn's is that there is a basic genetic fault in the mucous lining of the small intestine especially—it is too permeable. Certainly the permeability is increased when the illness is in an active phase.

One refinement that gives even better results with the diet is the inclusion of an antibiotic in the package. This is hedging the bets. Whether it is intolerance of certain foods or bacteria habitually living in the gut causing the symptoms, the diet-cum-drug treatment is bound to win.

Total Parenteral Nutrition (TPN)

In total parenteral nutrition all the nourishment is administered into a vein. Eight out of ten people with Crohn's go into remission on an elemental diet, and the results are similar with TPN. It used to be thought that both these diets were effective because they gave the bowel a rest from the physical work of pushing the part-digested food along its length. Liquid food simply percolates down.

However, a carefully restricted diet that includes solids can be just as successful—it is not the mechanical rest that benefits the intestines and allows them to recover. Perhaps the absence of particular foods has an effect on the bacteria that live in the gut because *their* diet is altered. It seems that whatever else, the diets are more likely to be beneficial if the proteins in them are converted to amino acids before they are eaten.

Mohammed

Mohammed had lived in Birmingham, England, since age three and had adopted a British lifestyle and eating habits. He fell victim to Crohn's, an illness of Western culture, when he was in his twenties. He suffered badly. Because of recurrent blockage of his small intestine and an alarming loss of weight, Mohammed's specialist advised him to have a fairly limited, unhealthy section of his ileum removed. Nevertheless he was worried that Mohammed would not have the resilience, despite his youth, to recover quickly from the surgery. It was important to him not to miss the final examinations for his computer studies.

Two weeks on an elemental diet had Mohammed ready to rebel against the regimen, but at least he was fitter and heavier than he had been for months. The operation went according to plan, and Mohammed was able to take his exam in June. He passed.

No one can stay on an elemental diet indefinitely, and although the symptoms subside—or remit—with the diet, they inevitably return, sooner rather than later, when the diet is stopped. One answer is to repeat the diet for a few weeks every time diarrhea or abdominal pain starts up again. At one clinic the patients have four weeks of elemental diet every four months, to renew the beneficial effects. However, it seems even better if you can find a diet you can live with long term—one that avoids the substances your body objects to. The essential thing is to know what these are and eliminate them.

ELIMINATION DIETS

Dr. Hunter found that more than three-quarters of his patients, who were all quite seriously ill to begin with, recovered after two to four weeks on the elemental diet, and then reacted to specific foods when these were introduced during an elimination diet later. If they avoided these particular foods most of them remained well for the next two years.

Elimination diets are a way of detecting the offenders in food intolerance, and they rid you of your symptoms for the duration as well. The diets comprise three stages:

- Exclusion—all the foods you eat normally are withdrawn.
- Reintroduction—foods are introduced one at a time.
- Refurbished eating habits, omitting the troublemakers.

The Exclusion Phase

The drawback of this phase is that you cannot have any food that you normally eat. It is a test of willpower.

Some doctors give their patients five days on nothing but bottled water as an exclusion period. This is not a viable plan in Crohn's, because you definitely need all the nourishment you can manage. Besides, it is such an abnormal step that your whole metabolism goes topsy-turvy, and this could upset your reactions in stage two.

If you do not need to go on an elemental diet, other exclusion diets are commonly used.

Pears and Lamb Diet: This or any other combination of an animal protein and a fruit or vegetable that you seldom eat. The point is to have something that your body has not dealt with often enough to develop a sensitivity.

Few Foods Diet: This provides you with a dozen rather than only two choices, but you must not pick your favorites. You must also miss:

- alcohol, coffee, tea (including herb tea), and sodas
- chocolate, sweets and candies, sugary foods, and artificial sweeteners
- vinegar, pickles, and highly spiced or salty foods
- take-out food, sausages, paté, curry, smoked fish, and ham
- restaurant meals

Your doctor or dietician can help you work out a selection that covers your body's needs. For example, you can have turnips instead of carrots, soft tofu rather than cottage cheese, rye bread instead of wheat, and so on.

Rare Foods Diet: This is one for the affluent eater. It means hunting for the exotic, such delicacies as paw-paw, truffles, caviar, tapioca, pomegranates, pine nuts, chickpeas (a good source of protein), goose, rabbit, venison, pumpkin, and pumpkin seeds.

A combination of rare and few foods diets is probably the most tolerable. The exclusion phase must run for three or four weeks, and that is a good time to get into the habit of jotting down in a daily diary what you eat and when, your Crohn's or other symptoms, and your mood. This will be vital for stage two.

If you are no better after two weeks on the exclusion diet, the next step is to try a more rigorous version, even an elemental diet. Stay on that for a month. It will not harm you—in fact, quite the reverse. It supplies all your body's needs in the easiest form for it to absorb. If you actually feel worse on whichever exclusion diet you chose, change to the elemental diet anyway—as treatment.

If you are improved but only slightly, it is probably worthwhile to stick with the diet you are on for the full month. There is no point in going on to stage two if you are not substantially better, but you have nothing to regret health-wise in having at least achieved the exclusion period.

The Reintroduction Phase

You may feel deprived after the weeks on the exclusion phase, but physically and nutritionally you will be improved after the first two weeks. Now you move into the positive part. You and your digestive system will meet old friends and sort out those that are not true friends but troublemakers. It takes seven or eight weeks to work through the reintroduction of foods you have excluded, spending two or three days on each. Try each food two days running and watch for any unpleasant reaction—Crohn's-type symptoms or headache, stomachache, feeling sick or faint, vomiting. In this phase the diary of foods, symptoms, and emotions becomes key. It is a record you should keep for future reference.

If food intolerance is an important feature in your Crohn's, there will probably be two or three foods that your body rejects. If you react to five or more, this is likely to be a food allergy, unrelated to Crohn's and requiring specific antiallergy treatment. When you have identified foodstuffs you must avoid, remember to look out for them in unexpected places, especially in gourmet cookery, where small amounts of numerous ingredients might be melded together or concealed in a delicious sauce—enough to confuse any taste bud.

Refurbishment Phase

This is the fun part. You rebuild your diet along healthy lines, scrupulously avoiding the elements that are bad for you. Aim toward the special Crohn's diet on page 156, with the emphasis on high protein, low fat, plenty of fruits and vegetables, and not too much of the very sweet. Foods you should include for sure (unless they are on your personal no-go list) are:

- whole-grain bread, potatoes, brown rice
- milk, butter (a little), simple cheeses
- cereals that have no added sugar, such as Shredded Wheat, Puffed Wheat
- oatmeal
- fresh, unprocessed meat
- fish (not smoked), especially tuna and salmon
- beans and lentils
- unsweetened fruit juice
- lots of fresh fruit—raw, stewed, or baked
- plenty of vegetables, especially green leafy ones and salads

Give your new, improved diet a month, then take stock, and adjust it as necessary within the guidelines. When you have carefully avoided a particular food for six months or more—preferably a year—it is worth trying cautiously to find out whether your sensitivity to it has faded. Take small amounts only.

Rebecca

Rebecca was widowed at 43, and within the next three months developed arthritis. Fortunately, her children, Paul and Becky, were old enough to help when their mother's joints were particularly stiff and painful. The symptoms of

Crohn's disease came on almost imperceptibly at the same time. To wake herself up and hopefully pep up her energy Rebecca had taken to drinking "gallons" of coffee. She had probably sensitized herself to it, but just cutting that down had no appreciable effect. The doctor was worried about Rebecca's loss of weight—ten pounds in six weeks seemed too much to be accounted for by the bereavement.

The hospital tests gave the answer: Crohn's disease. Drinking nourishing supplements made very little difference to Rebecca's weight, and her abdominal pain and the diarrhea continued. The doctor gave her a choice—to go on steroids or put up with an elemental diet as an introduction to an elimination study. She decided on the diet, encouraged by Paul and Becky, and over the next few weeks she began to feel better, both in the Crohn's symptoms and the arthritis. She regained several pounds. The second phase of the elimination process showed that coffee and tomatoes were foods she needed to avoid.

She is now well into remission, including abatement of the arthritic pains. She is now a tea and fruit-juice drinker. No tomatoes.

Chapter 12

Eating Well

Eating well is an indispensable part of health and happy living, and for those with Crohn's it is doubly important.
Unlike the 35 percent of the population of the United
States who are currently obsessed with shedding weight, Crohn's
patients need every calorie they can get. It is not just quantity but
quality the body requires. Crohn's sufferers cannot afford to bur-
den their sensitive digestive systems with junk foods and irritants;
they have a special need for vitamins and essential minerals.
Although patients are sure to be taking some supplements, it is
wise to take the foods in which they occur naturally as well, for
maximum absorption.

WHY CROHN'S PATIENTS SHOULD
EAT BETTER THAN OTHER PEOPLE

1. A poor appetite—anorexia—is a common symptom of
   Crohn's disease, often one of the earliest and most pervasive.
   It means that there are periods when your intake is very
   small, so that what you eat must be especially nutritious.

2. An essential feature of Crohn's is damage, through inflammation, of the mucous lining of the digestive system. This
   interferes with both the digestion of your food and its
   absorption.

3. The digestion of fats in the upper parts of the small intestine is often only half-completed, and this has secondary adverse effects. Part-digested fat arriving in the ileum, lower down, cannot be absorbed but clogs up the delicate, specialized lining membrane. All absorption is further impaired. Pale, copious stools are a sign that too much fat is being passed out, undigested, with the waste.

4. Inflammation and ulceration of the ileum, the typical result of Crohn's, prevents it from carrying out its function of absorption. This applies not only to the basic food elements—proteins, carbohydrates, and fats—but crucially to the essential vitamins and minerals without which the rest of our food is worthless.

5. The digestion and absorption of starchy foods—that is, all the carbohydrates except sugar—is diminished because of the effect of Crohn's on the jejunum, which runs into the ileum. Carbohydrates comprise the bulk of our food.

6. If the colon is affected by Crohn's there is an extra loss of minerals. They are carried away dissolved in an excess of water that would normally have been salvaged by the absorptive part of the colon.

7. In an acute phase the patient may lose nourishment directly, through vomiting.

8. Diarrhea means that part-digested foods are washed away down the toilet.

9. While you have an active inflammatory process going on, including a degree of fever, you burn up your food faster.

10. Protein-losing enteropathy: when the intestines are healthy, they throw off a lot of protein with discarded cells, since they are constantly renewing their lining. When they are irritated or inflamed this process is enormously increased, and the small intestine in particular pours out water and valuable protein. You can easily drink water, but replacing protein requires serious eating.

11. Postoperative states: if you have surgery to remove diseased segments of the small intestine you may be left with a restricted amount of absorptive mucous membrane. If you have an ileostomy or a colostomy, especially the former, you will lose some of your fairly well digested food, plus water, salt, and other minerals. They literally go to waste.

12. Undernutrition itself, since it also starves the digestive system, impairs both digestion and absorption and causes or increases diarrhea. It can lead to a shortage of the trace metal zinc.

13. Zinc deficiency reduces your intake because it makes food seem less attractive. There is a loss of the sense of smell, *hyposmia*, and of taste, *hypogeusia*.

14. Emotional disturbance: depression and anxiety are understandably common in Crohn's. Depression kills the appetite, and anxiety disturbs the digestion and by increasing muscle tension increases the demand for fuel.

UNDERNUTRITION

With all these reasons for an inadequate food intake and an inability to make full use of it, it is no wonder that undernutrition is one of the cardinal symptoms of Crohn's. Some of its effects, apart from the vicious circle of the worsening of digestion and absorption, include:

- weight loss
- feeling tired all the time
- low physical energy
- low mental energy, showing up as poor concentration and memory
- muscle weakness
- anemia
- lack of protein

- feeling cold
- difficulty in shaking off colds, and slow healing of minor injuries

Other symptoms and signs might alert you to a deficiency of vitamins or minerals, in particular:

- mouth ulcers
- cracks in the skin by your nails and the corners of your mouth
- pale skin and membranes in your mouth or lower eyelid
- dry, parched skin
- bruises appearing with little or no cause
- ridges on your nails
- brittle, splitting nails
- sore tongue
- thinning hair

The effects of specific vitamin and mineral deficiencies are described in chapter 3. If you have any of these signs and symptoms, see your doctor for a checkup—vitamins and minerals matter enormously to your health.

WHAT TO EAT TO PROVIDE THE VITAMINS YOU NEED

Vitamin A

This comes in two forms: retinol, the vitamin itself, which is fat-soluble and comes from animal sources; and beta-carotene, a pro-vitamin that your body converts into the vitamin as needed. Over-dosing on vitamin A is dangerous—Sir Ranulph Fiennes nearly killed himself by eating too much liver on a polar expedition, and there is a government health warning advising pregnant women against eating liver. The liver stores vitamin A. Beta-carotene comes from plants and carries no risks because it is water-soluble and the body passes out what it does not need through the urine.

Both vitamin A and beta-carotene are antioxidants (see below), and their advantages include a protective influence against some cancers and anti-infective properties for the skin and membranes.

Where to Find Beta-Carotene

- carrots and dark green, leafy vegetables such as spinach and broccoli

- melons, apricots, pumpkins

These also supply fiber and vitamin C.

Where to Find Vitamin A

- liver (but don't overdo it)

- dairy products, eggs

- salmon, sardines, tuna, fish oils

The vitamin itself is not destroyed by cooking, unlike beta-carotene.

Supplements: A special supplement of vitamin A is rarely necessary unless you have Crohn's; most people need beta-carotene capsules only if they are unable to eat any vegetables or fruit.

Fish oils contain *eicosapentanoeic acid*—EPA for simplicity— one of the essential fatty acids in the Omega-3 group. This has major anti-inflammatory powers, and some research studies have reported remarkably good results in over half the cases of Crohn's disease. Instead of the capsules, you can take that well-established standby, cod liver oil, or eat one or two meals a week that include oily fish. Plant sources of Omega-3, such as flaxseed oil, hemp oil, evening primrose oil, and blackcurrant oil, do not contain EPA.

Vitamin D (Calciferol)

Like vitamin A, this is oil- or fat-based, an antioxidant, and not destroyed by cooking. It is needed for the absorption of calcium and zinc, but itself increases the demand for magnesium.

Where to Find It

- oily fish (the carnivorous group): sardines, herring, mackerel, salmon, pilchards

- margarine (always has vitamins A and D added), eggs, liver

Sunlight on the skin enables us to make our own vitamin D, but dark-skinned people living in northern latitudes are at a disadvantage. The pale northern rays do not get through.

Supplements: Cod-liver or other fish oil by spoon or capsule—see under vitamin A. With Crohn's you need to take a fish oil or eat oily fish regularly, but overdosage can occur. Get medical advice if you are pregnant or might be.

Vitamin E (Tocopherol)

This is also oily and occurs both in fish oils and plants. It is another antioxidant (see below). Because with Crohn's your digestive system may be inefficient in absorbing fats, you may require extra vitamin E. It is still controversial whether it has any useful role, but it has been suggested as helpful in a dozen disorders from infertility to diabetes.

Where to Find It

- wheat germ and other vegetable oils
- whole-grain bread and cereals
- butter and margarine
- eggs and broccoli

It does not stand up to heating or refrigeration.

Supplements: Capsules or tablets, including the chewable variety. The USDA suggests 3–4 mg as a suitable dose, but there are no agreed signs or symptoms of vitamin E deficiency.

Antioxidants

Antioxidants comprise a group of unrelated chemical substances that protect the tissues, to some extent, from the effects of *free rad-icals*. These are especially reactive atoms or compounds, also called oxidants, that hasten the damaging effects of aging, degenerative diseases, and any chronic disorder. A sufficiency of antioxidants is especially desirable in Crohn's and helps to prevent the development of cancer in later life. Vitamins A, C, and E, and beta-carotene are all important antioxidants.

Vitamin B1 (Thiamin)

The whole complex of B vitamins is associated with digestion. Vitamin B1 is water-soluble, which means that it is lost when vegetables or fruit are cooked in water. High-temperature cooking like roasting, grilling, and frying and also the canning process destroy it. Potatoes baked in their jackets lose their thiamin, but boiled in their skins they keep most of it. Preservatives and baking powder destroy it, and even chopping, mincing, or liquidizing the food means the loss of three-quarters of the vitamin.

Where to Find It

- Luckily that staple food, whole-grain bread, is an excellent source—so long as you do not toast it.

- Other whole-grain cereals, wheat germ, pasta, rice, and yeast.

- Kidneys, liver, and pork.

There is no risk from accidental overdose, since any surplus is disposed of in the urine, but it reacts with *levodopa*, a medicine for Parkinson's disease. You can run short of thiamin because of poor absorption from the small intestine or if you drink alcohol in excess. It is worth ensuring an adequate supply because it appears to have a beneficial effect on the intestines since it speeds up recovery from gastroenteritis.

Supplements: A daily compound vitamin B tablet will supply all you need.

Vitamin B2 (Riboflavin)

This vitamin contributes to the digestion and efficient usage of both carbohydrates and proteins, and it facilitates the absorption of iron, vitamin B6, and folate. It stands up quite well to cooking, but deteriorates if exposed to sunlight—the milk bottle left on the doorstep all day. This does not matter to most people, because it is found in a wide variety of foods, but with Crohn's you need to make sure that you have enough of this important vitamin.

Where to Find It

- milk and cheese (the main sources)
- liver, kidney, eggs, wheat germ and bran, cereals with commercially added vitamins

Supplements: A daily B-complex tablet is likely to be sufficient. The minimum dose is 1 mg daily, but you will require 3–4 mg, plus extra if you are taking a tricyclic antidepressant such as amitriptyline, or the tranquilizer chlorpromazine. Overdosage is not a danger.

Lack of riboflavin is reputed to be the cause of cracks in the corners of the mouth and a sore, red tongue, but other conditions, for instance a shortage of niacin, vitamin C, or iron, may be responsible.

Vitamin B3 (Niacin, Nicotinic Acid)

This stimulates your circulation and helps with chilblains and menstrual cramps. It also makes your skin feel hot. You must not take it in tablet form if you have a peptic ulcer.

Where to Find It

- yeast, peanuts, bran
- whole grains, coffee
- liver, kidney, meat, fish

Supplements: Again, the B-complex tablet will include enough niacin.

Vitamin B6 (Pyridoxine)

B6 is necessary for amino-acid metabolism, enabling you to make the best use of your proteins—something you are likely to lack. It also has a beneficial effect on mood, especially the depression sometimes associated with taking estrogens, found in birth-control pills or hormone replacement therapy.

Where to Find It

- liver, kidneys, meat, fish, eggs
- whole-grain cereals, potatoes
- bananas, avocados, walnuts,

It will survive gentle cooking.

Vitamin B12 (Cobalamin)

This was not isolated until 1948. Before that people like George Bernard Shaw, who suffered from a serious form of anemia, had to eat large quantities of liver. Now cobalamin can be given by injection. The related anemia that arises in Crohn's is due to the failure of the small intestine to absorb this vitamin and its partner, folic acid. There is a very high risk of B12 supplies falling short after surgery to remove diseased parts of the ileum. The treatment of this anemia is the same as for Shaw's pernicious type: regular injections every three months.

Where to Find It

- liver, kidney, sardines, oysters, meat
- eggs, cheese, milk

Because it is found in animal sources only, vegans are highly susceptible to a dangerous B12 deficiency, with physical and mental symptoms. A diet that excludes meat is unsafe in Crohn's (see chapter 3).

Folic Acid, Folates

This vitamin gets its name from *foliage*, the leaves of a plant, because that is where you find it. It works in collaboration with vitamin B12 in the manufacturing and maturing of red blood corpuscles in the bone marrow. The two are also involved in the production of DNA, the blueprint chemical for your whole body. A lack of folate brings on all the anemic and other symptoms of B12 deficiency. Folic acid is particularly important in pregnancy.

Where to Find It

- green leafy vegetables, lettuce, and beets

- oranges, bananas, and avocados

- whole-grain bread, bran, eggs, and uncooked peanuts

Supplements: A daily tablet ensures an adequate supply. There is no overdosage problem.

Vitamin C (Ascorbic Acid)

This is another antioxidant that hopefully protects the tissues, including those of the digestive system, from succumbing too fast to wear and tear. Injuries and Crohn's ulcers heal better with plenty of vitamin C, and in the treatment of anemia it helps the absorption of iron. Plenty does not mean megadoses, however, since they can lead to withdrawal symptoms.

We do not see scurvy these days, but a shortage of vitamin C shows itself by spontaneous bruising, anemia, and spongy, friable gums. People in hospitals or other institutions where there is mass cooking are often short of vitamin C; it can be cooked away, and fresh foods tend to be a rarity in such places.

Where to Find It

- strawberries, citrus fruits, guavas and other tropical fruits

- green peppers, salad vegetables (raw)
- vegetables of the brassica group: cabbage, broccoli, sprouts, cauliflower—as crudités or lightly cooked
- potatoes, milk

It is quickly destroyed by cooking, exposure to the air, and by cutting, peeling, and washing.

Supplements: Since your body can neither make this vitamin nor store it, it is sensible to make sure of your daily intake, in winter especially, by taking a daily tablet. Even if you are not anemic—but more so if you are—vitamin C gives a boost to your feeling of energy.

Unfortunately several medicines work against vitamin C, including steroids, which are very relevant to Crohn's; also aspirin, tetracycline, and indomethacin.

Vitamin K

The "K" comes from the word for coagulation in Danish, because this vitamin is necessary for the blood to clot. It comes in two forms: K1 and K2. K1 can be lacking in Crohn's through poor absorption, and K2 because of a change of bacteria in the colon from the illness.

Where to Find It

- green, leafy vegetables like spinach
- cauliflower
- alfalfa
- it may be manufactured in the colon by some friendly strains of E. coli

Supplements

- If a clotting time test shows that you are low in vitamin K, which could lead to severe bleeding from ulcerated areas, tablets or injections are available.

MINERALS

Some chemicals play an important role in the structure and functioning of the body—think of iron in the blood and calcium in the bones. Only very small amounts are required, but they are absolutely vital. The Crohn's sufferer is in a vulnerable situation because of the double whammy of poor absorption and extra losses through the bowels.

Calcium

This is important for the health and strength of bones and teeth, especially in children and the elderly. Children with Crohn's are in danger of poor, stunted growth, particularly affecting the long bones—adequate supplies of calcium are vital. Pregnant women need extra supplies, and from middle age onward there is the specter of osteoporosis. Calcium is also involved in the nerves supplying the muscles. Everyone needs vitamin D to be able to absorb calcium, especially the vulnerable groups including people with Crohn's or anorexia nervosa.

Where to Find It

- cheese, milk, yogurt
- fish eaten with the bones: sardines, pilchards, canned salmon
- peanuts, almonds, chickpeas, beans
- eggs, bread to which calcium has been added (see *Phytates*, below)

Iron

Iron is an essential ingredient of hemoglobin, the oxygen-carrying compound in red blood cells. It is so precious that it is salvaged and recycled by the body—but in Crohn's it is poorly absorbed and often lost in the stools from diarrhea. Iron-deficiency anemia is so common as to be almost standard in Crohn's (see page 56).

Where to Find It

- meat, poultry, liver, fish (especially sardines), eggs
- whole-grain cereals, oatmeal, All-Bran (see *Phytates*, below)
- peas, beans, lentils, spinach
- prunes, raisins
- chocolate

Vitamin C enhances the absorption of iron, but tea and coffee inhibit it. Vegetarians, even without Crohn's, often become iron-deficient, and should never drink tea or coffee with their meals. If you are a Crohn's sufferer it is vital not to restrict your diet.

Supplements: You probably need to take iron tablets anyway, but will for sure if you have either type of anemia. In some people they cause pain and disturbance of the intestines, either constipation or diarrhea, but there are several different preparations, one of which might suit you.

Magnesium

This is necessary for the health of the brain and nerves. A lack of it can cause depression, agitation, or confusion. You can run short of magnesium in Crohn's because of general undernutrition, diarrhea, or vomiting.

Where to Find It

- cocoa, plain chocolate
- cashews, almonds, brazil nuts
- shrimps and prawns
- barley, wheat, peas, beans

Supplements: You can buy tablets in natural-food stores, but it is better to take it in your diet (see *Phytates*, below).

Zinc

Zinc deficiency was first recognized in 1972, and it is now established that the absence of the tiny amount the body needs can cause far-reaching effects. These include diarrhea, mental apathy, weakness of the muscles, nerve pain, and a loss of the senses of smell and taste.

Where to Find It

- oysters, sardines
- meat and liver
- whole grains, oatmeal, breakfast cereals
- nuts, peas, beans

Supplements: Zinc can run short in Crohn's sufferers from malabsorption and losses in the stool. Tablets may be used to ensure an intake of 15 mg a day (see *Phytates*, below).

Selenium

This is another antioxidant and can be beneficial in Crohn's. Its action is related to that of vitamin E, but little else is known about it.

Where to Find It

- Whole-grain bread and other whole-grain foods, especially if they come from grain grown in America (European soil contains very little selenium).
- Brazil nuts

Supplements: Tablets are available in health stores, but there is little reason to suppose they will benefit you.

Phytic Acid, Phytates

If you pride yourself on a healthy diet, never eating white bread or sugared cereal, but whole-grain everything from bread to tortillas to pasta, oats for breakfast as porridge or granola, and bran scattered on top, you will be in fashion. You may also be depriving your body of some essential minerals. Simply using plenty of bran because it is "good for you" cause serious mineral deficiencies, because of the phytates in it.

They do their damage by latching on to iron, calcium, zinc, and magnesium and forming insoluble compounds that cannot be absorbed and are passed out with the stool. Fortunately, whole-grain *bread* retains its iron and calcium in particular, because the yeast in it counteracts the phytate. And you can make a (health) case for eating phytate-free white bread whenever you fancy a change.

FIBER

This is a food that provides us with no nourishment yet it is necessary to our health, especially that of the small and large intestines. Its value was first brought to common notice by an Englishman, Dr. T. R. Allinson, and two Americans, Dr. John Harvey Kellogg and the philanthropist Sylvester Graham. Graham crackers were developed as a kind of digestive biscuit.

An earlier term was *roughage*, then came *fiber*, and since the early 1990s the British Department of Health has said:

- We should have more of it;

- We should call it *non-starch polysaccharides*—NSP for short.

I prefer the term fiber. In essence it comprises all the parts of a plant that we cannot digest. There are several different sorts, for example, pectin, cellulose, hemicellulose, and lignin. They are all carbohydrates. Their most remarkable feature is their ability to absorb water—15 times their own weight. This makes for a stool that is firm but soft and that causes no irritation as it passes down the gut. It also increases the bulk of the stool.

Fiber is particularly beneficial in Crohn's, when poor appetite and impaired functioning of the gut may produce a stool that is too little and too liquid to stimulate movement or to control.

Our current preference for highly refined, processed foods— white bread, cakes and sweet rolls, white rice, and sugar as pure, white sucrose—deprive the small and large intestines of the exercise they need to keep fit. A low-fiber diet can lead to constipation in the short term, but more seriously and insidiously, over time, to diverticular disease, gallstones, irritable colon, and ultimately colon cancer.

The recommended intake of fiber should be between 12 and 32 grams daily (32 g is a little over an ounce—not much).

Where to Find It

- bran, bran cereals like All-Bran

- whole grains, oatmeal, brown rice

- dried fruit, especially prunes

- potatoes in their jackets, especially the jackets

- raw, fresh fruit, especially bananas

- salads, green vegetables, nuts

By far the best source is bran, either wheat or oat. The latter is preferable because it contains less phytate. This means that not as much of the minerals iron, calcium, zinc, and magnesium is made unabsorbable (see *Phytates*, above). A test of whether you are eating enough fiber is to check whether your stool sinks like a stone in the toilet or tends to float. Fiber is light.

Some high-fiber foods may cause gas indigestion. An excess of gas is produced in the colon, causing pain and bloating. Taking iron pills—usually for anemia—sometimes alleviates the situation.

THE IMMUNE SYSTEM

Since the immune system is your main defense against the enemies of the body, including any sneaky bugs that are involved in Crohn's disease, it is essential to supply it with the fuel it needs.

The Organization of the Immune System

The immune system accounts for 2 percent of your body weight—the same amount as your brain. It consists of cells produced in the bone marrow, some of which travel all over your body—a mobile fighting force—while others aggregate together in lymph glands. Some are dispersed between other cells in the lining of intestine.

The immune cells come in two major families, the Ts and the Bs.

The T Cells

- *T helper cells* assess the dangers and switch on the immune system when necessary. These cells are knocked out by the AIDS virus.

- *T suppressor cells* switch the system off when the attack is over.

- *T cytotoxic cells* are killers—of cancer cells and other undesirables.

- *T DTH cells* mediate delayed hypersensitivity, which may be relevant to reactions to food or bacteria in Crohn's disease.

T cells are able to cope with bacteria, fungi, and viruses that get inside healthy cells.

The B Lymphocytes

These cells make up the mobile fighting force that homes in on trouble spots, such as patches of Crohn's, an injury, or an infection. There are several types.

- *Polymorphonuclear granulocytes* (polymorphs for short): they kill and eat invaders. People who run short of these are pushovers for infections.

- *Macrophages:* polymorphs are small but macrophages are large (macro = big), and they swallow up germs of all types and also cancer cells. They lurk around in the vicinity of an infection, inflammation, or tumor. As well as attacking the bad guys, they trigger local blood-clotting and are instrumental in the repair and remodeling of damaged tissues.

- *NK (natural killer) cells:* their special mission is to root out viruses and destroy them.

The B cells produce antibodies, chemical substances called immunoglobulins. These come in different classes—IgG (Immunoglobulin G) is the most common. They deal with specific enemies. For instance they immobilize the diphtheria germ so that a polymorph or macrophage can gobble it up. IgA (Immunoglobulin A) specializes in gut problems. It confers a measure of immunity to unfriendly bacteria and can sort out the good from the bad.

WHAT THE IMMUNE SYSTEM NEEDS

Minerals

- *Calcium* is needed by the macrophages and polymorphs in particular, and works in conjunction with magnesium. Root vegetables are the best source of magnesium.

- *Iron* boosts overall resistance to infection. Too much in concentrated form can be toxic, so try to get all you can through your food, helped by vitamin C.

- *Zinc and selenium* are both useful antioxidants. Zinc is needed in the maturation of T cells and selenium in antibody production.

Vitamins

- *Vitamin A* is particularly effective where there is a high risk of infection, such as the nose and throat, the genital and urinary areas, and the bowels. It is used in the production of *lysozyme*, an antibacterial enzyme found in tears, sweat, saliva, and other body fluids.

- *B-complex vitamins*, especially B12 and folic acid, are involved in all types of healing—including that of Crohn's ulcers—and of growth in the young. B6, pyridoxine, is used by the cells that eat up invaders.

- *Vitamin C* slows down the rate of multiplication of most viruses and boosts the production of both T and B leukocytes.

IMMUNE-SYSTEM SUPPRESSORS

Obviously, after an infection or other attack on the body has passed or healed, you do not need the immune system working at full blast. It would be like having the central heating on full blast in midsummer. The T suppressor cells switch it off as needed, but some other substances and some circumstances suppress the immune system just when you need it. They include:

- Vitamin D in excess.

- Coffee, tea, and other stimulants (speed, cocaine, Ecstasy).

- Alcohol and marijuana. Both of these first briefly stimulate then suppress the immune system. This mirrors the psychological effect of drinking—you are happy and witty after the first glass but as you take more you function less efficiently.

- Missing a whole night's sleep (alternately drowsing and waking all night does not count).

- Chronic stress, leading to irritability and pessimism.

- Lack of fresh air, exercise, or social contacts.

- Lack of an intimate relationship, including sex.

- Breathing polluted air—exhausting for your immune system.

Contrary to the stereotype of a boring, colorless health-food regimen, a wholesome and satisfying diet permits many positive options for anyone aiming to prevent or treat Crohn's disease. From the lists in this chapter and the guidelines offered in the next, you and your doctor or dietician can personalize an eating plan that is well suited for you—and is sure to appeal to your taste buds, too.

Chapter 13

Constructing Your Personal Diet

The diet that will serve you and your body best will depend on the state of your Crohn's disease and your personal situation at the time.

- Is the illness active, recovering, or in remission?

- Have you a stoma to consider, after an ostomy?

- Are you pregnant?

- Are you still growing?

- Are you under any particular stress?

The mix of nourishment most likely to keep you well during remission, or to aim toward after a bad period, includes many of the elements of an anticancer diet. The cornerstones are proteins, carbohydrates, and fats, and in Crohn's you need all the trimmings— vitamins, minerals, and fiber. You need more calories than other people do, so do not hold back, on proteins especially, and carbohydrates, but be careful with fats and highly refined sugar.

First and most important—you must enjoy your meals. A poor appetite is one of the main problems in Crohn's. Here are some general guidelines.

- Aim for pleasant surroundings and pleasant company, and when you are at home make your table or tray look attractive.

- Allow plenty of time to eat, and slow the pace by reading a book if you are by yourself. Slowing down helps your digestive system by allowing you to chew each mouthful properly, it also enables you to appreciate flavors to the full.

- Choose simple foods, but of the top quality. It is false economy to treat your body to second best when food is fundamental to your health.

SPECIAL CIRCUMSTANCES

Pregnancy

If your Crohn's is inactive, avoid liver, lightly cooked eggs, and cheeses other than cottage cheese or cheddar, and be sure to have foods that contain all the vitamins and essential minerals. Folate is especially important, and you need a supplement, probably a multivitamin-and-mineral type. Babies are built on protein, so make sure you have your daily quota.

If your Crohn's is acting up, a formula diet, including an elemental, is safe and particularly effective in pregnancy.

Children and Adolescents

Young children who are not growing at a satisfactory rate may need to have a course of tube feeding to get the extra nutrition they need. An adolescent who is behind in height or sexual development also urgently requires a boost. An elemental or less severe formula diet, by tube if necessary, will save him or her from permanently stunted growth and reproductive immaturity. Calcium with vitamin D is needed for growing bones—and again, they need plenty of protein. This is not the time to turn vegetarian, since it is difficult to eat enough legumes and grains to supply vegetarian protein—apart from the need for vitamin B12, which comes only from animal sources.

With an Ileostomy or Colostomy

Normally the colon absorbs a liter of water a day. After these operations it is no longer available to reabsorb water and the essential minerals dissolved in it. After an ileostomy, it is not only the scarce minerals such as iron and magnesium that need replacing, you also lose a great deal of salt (sodium chloride). Both fluid and minerals, especially salt, must be made up, and supplements are necessary. Ileostomy diarrhea is a common complication that intensifies the problem.

The significant improvements in how you feel a few months after an ostomy are well worth the few adjustments you need to make in your diet.

Diarrhea

This symptom is likely to occur from time to time, or it may be a long-term tendency in your case. In the acute stage you may be restricted to plenty of such drinks as very weak tea, with dry toast or melba toast. In the recovery phase, or if you are often prone to diarrhea, you should have:

- small, frequent meals

- smooth, unstimulating food without condiments, spices, or pickles

- nothing very hot or refrigerated

- plenty to drink, especially between meals

- adequate protein, B-complex vitamins, and vitamin C

Avoid:

- alcohol, strong tea, or coffee

- meat extracts

- fried food

- fresh bread or hot buttered toast

- sausages, bacon, pork, twice-cooked meat, visible fat on meat

- unripe or dried fruit

BLAND DIET

A bland diet may be called for when you are recovering from an attack and need to build up gently. The following can serve as a guideline:

On waking
Weak tea with milk and sugar
Dry toast or melba toast

Breakfast
Strained porridge with milk and pureed fruit
Egg or a tiny portion of steamed white fish
Crisp toast, spread when cold
Runny honey, jelly, or golden syrup

Mid-morning
Milky drink, banana, or plain crackers

Lunch
Fish, lean, tender meat or chicken, or soft cheese
Puréed vegetables, e.g., broccoli and carrots, plus mashed potatoes, pasta, or crisp toast
Yogurt, cottage cheese, or rice pudding with puréed fruit, applesauce, or stewed or baked apple
Diluted fruit drink

Late afternoon
Crisp toast, spread when cold and split into sandwiches with a soft-boiled egg or soft cheese, or with honey or jelly
Plain cake crackers
Weak tea

Supper
As lunch, with weak coffee afterwards, if desired

Late evening
Small milky drink
Sliced banana

DIET FOR GENERAL USE
WITH CROHN'S DISEASE

When the symptoms are not troublesome or you are in complete remission, the guiding principle is high protein and low fat.
Points to note:

1. Protein is the build-and-repair food. Twice a day have a protein meal, with meat, fish, egg, or cheese as the main ingredient in at least one. For the other, choose vegetable proteins with legumes and grains, tofu or tempeh (a fermented soy product similar to tofu), or nuts. The disadvantages of vegetarian foods are that they do not supply vitamin B12 (essential), and it is difficult to take in enough calories, especially since you cannot have extra fat.

2. Once or twice a week have fish, preferably salmon, sardine, herring, tuna, mackerel, or shark.

3. Carbohydrates, the energy foods, supply the bulk of your diet, but beware of refined sugar, refined flour products, or white rice. Alcohol counts as sugar.

4. Fats and oils: fish oil from the fatty fish listed above is especially beneficial in Crohn's, but be sparing with other fats.

5. Fiber is another food particularly useful in Crohn's. Choose, by trial and error, which type is least likely to give you excess gas, especially if you have a stoma. Eat plenty of fruits and vegetables, either raw or nearly so. Pick whole-grain bread, pasta, and spaghetti.

6. If you must cook, microwave, steam, grill, or bake in foil.

7. *Rarely* have a burger, luncheon meat, sausages, processed ham, cakes, biscuits, ice cream, or pizza.

8. Remember, you are trying to maintain or increase your weight.

HIGH-PROTEIN, LOW-FAT
GENERAL PURPOSE DIET

On waking
Tea or fruit juice

Breakfast
Fruit juice (optional)
Cereal with fresh or stewed fruit
Egg, sardine, slice of cheese or ham, tomato
Whole-grain toast with margarine, honey, or marmalade
Coffee, tea, or low-fat chocolate

Mid-morning
Drink as above and/or piece of fruit

Lunch
Meat, fish, egg, or cheese with salad or two vegetables, or baked
    potato or whole-grain bread sandwich filled with any of the
    above, plus a side salad
    or
Vegetable soup with whole-grain bread, if there is protein at two
    other meals
Fresh or stewed fruit or baked apple with yogurt, rice pudding and
    fruit
Herb tea, fruit drink, or mineral water
Coffee—not too often in the day or too strong

Late afternoon
Sandwich, or oat cake/rice cake and cheese
Fresh fruit
Drink as above

Supper
Soup (optional)
Meat, fish, egg, or cheese dish, plus two vegetables as well as pota-
    toes, brown rice, whole-grain roll, or pasta
    Fresh fruit, cheese, cookie or yogurt

Glass of wine, preferably white
Herb tea, coffee, or black tea

Late evening
Small hot drink, and a piece of fruit or a cookie if you wish
Follow this with enough sleep to wake refreshed.

Don't let yourself feel restricted by these suggestions—try as many options as possible from the huge variety of fruits and vegetables available in supermarkets these days, from all the corners of the earth. Sample all the different types of bread and forms of pasta. You need to experiment more conservatively only with the serious protein foods.

Bon appetit—and live well!

Chapter 14

Feeling and Coping:
The Psychological Aspects

A diagnosis of Crohn's disease is a watershed in your life, a moment of truth. Nothing will ever be quite the same again. It may hit you in one of three ways:

- Shock and disbelief—suddenly you are a person with a serious disorder.

- Heart-sinking confirmation of what you had suspected for some time; the only difference is that now it has a label.

- Relief at sharing the problem and having an ally in dealing with it.

After the initial impact, an avalanche of thoughts and questions comes tumbling into your mind:

- Why me? Is it anything I've done?

- It isn't fair.

- What will happen next? Will I get better? Could I die?

- What will happen to my job? How much time off will I need?

- Will my physical condition interfere with what I do?

- What will the treatment be like? Is it painful? Will I need to have an operation? (This is usually the time when horror stories come to mind about a distant cousin or someone's friend who had a bowel problem that might have been Crohn's.)

- How will my partner feel about my having a serious illness? Will it ruin the relationship?

- How will the rest of the family react? What will I tell them?

- What will it do to my sex life? If a man, will I be impotent? If a woman, will I still be attractive? Will I be able to have a baby?

- What happens if I have to rush to the toilet at a crucial time?

- What will my friends think? How will I explain?

The hardest part is usually the blow to your self-confidence, especially if you have always taken your body and its efficient functioning for granted. There is nothing dignified, let alone romantic, about an illness that affects the bowels. All the crude remarks using "asshole," "shit," and "up yours" jump out at you with new significance.

You may feel you are losing control, not only of your bowels but also of your life. This feeling is only temporary, while you find the best way, for you, of coming to grips with the situation. There are several tried and true methods of coping with adversity:

1. Forced optimism—denying that there is anything seriously wrong. "Just a touch of gastric flu," you may say, or "It's nothing to worry about"—although you are feeling dreadful. This natural reaction can help to carry you through the first shock while your mind adjusts to the reality. The danger is that it may lead you into refusing to get the treatment you need.

2. The opposite—passive acceptance and stoicism, which amount to pessimism. "What will be, will be," or "It's no good fighting against it," or even, "It's God's will." This is

definitely the worst attitude to any problem. You are pro-gramming yourself for invalidism.

3. Anger and resentment—this is better than pessimism, but you are wasting your energy. There is nothing constructive about such negative feelings, and it is a snub to the many people—friends, loved ones, professionals, and acquain-tances—who want to give you their support if you will let them.

4. Allowing yourself to become dependent, leaving the effort, the decisions, and the responsibility to others. This sce-nario gives you no goals, nothing to work for, nothing more inspiring to look forward to than lunch.

5. Taking on the real enemy—the illness—with all the courage and determination you can gather. You know this makes the most sense. Decide now that you are going to do whatever it takes to beat Crohn's disease, and you are not going to let it rob you of what you value most in life. Take time to review the things you value now, including:

- Relationships with the people who matter to you.

- Contributing to the well-being and happiness of people around you. This does wonders for your feelings of self-worth.

- Independence combined with graceful acceptance of the situation, including not being too proud to ask for help when you need it. People love to be of help.

- Making *new* friends and developing *new* interests. Treat life as an escalator.

WHAT SORT OF PEOPLE GET CROHN'S DISEASE?

The right answer is the unlucky ones. They are in every job or pro-fession—music, accounting, medicine, waiting tables, earning $20,000 or $200,000. If people are alike in being susceptible to the same bug or illness, there is a theory that they may be similar psychologically. Each of us is a unique, irreplaceable individual, but nevertheless people with Crohn's are more likely than average to be reliable and responsible, but not bossy—good colleagues to work with or to have as friends. A common trait is self-control, not complaining until they absolutely have to, and bottling up their feelings.

People with Crohn's are not typically the sort to throw their arms around you when they are happy or weep on your shoulder when they feel bad. They tend to dislike fuss and conflict and prefer to avoid confrontation.

This may not be you at all. If you have an easy, relaxed attitude toward life and are a natural communicator, be glad. If, on the other hand, you seldom display your feelings even when there is something on your mind as momentous as having Crohn's, other people will not guess what you are going through. Overcome your inhibitions and tell them of your anxiety, dismay, and sense of unfairness, or simply ask questions, and it will relieve the tension. Pent up emotions make pains and cramps worse, and unrelieved anxiety brings on diarrhea. Negative emotions act directly on your immune system, suppressing it. So, on a purely practical, physical basis, you need to unload the feelings that can disable your body's defenses.

COMMUNICATION IS THE KEY

You are not unusual if you find it difficult to talk with doctors and nurses—especially doctors—about what you want to know, or how you feel. More than 70 percent of people find it a problem, and the chief inhibition is usually that they are afraid they will sound foolish. Most doctors and nurses are not unsympathetic, but often they do not have the answers you expect them to have. Other common difficulties are:

- Not remembering later what the doctor said, particularly after the first, most important consultation, and then being reluctant to ask. Maybe you did not ask a question because you were afraid of what the answer might be—and now you wish you had.

- Not expressing your anxiety, depression, or confusion, or that you are "illogically" ashamed of the illness.

- Not asking details about the treatment—what it will do and whether it has side effects.

- Not asking whether you are improving medically.

If it is difficult talking with health professionals, it is no better with friends and relatives. What do you say when they tell you how much better you are looking, when you are feeling dreadful? Some of them visit you because of the illness but talk about everything else, while others are curious about the aspects you would rather not discuss. Some stay too long and wear you out, but these are minor things.

With the medical staff, be straightforward and determined—get your questions out or say what you feel at the first opportunity. With friends and relatives, use tact. The situation is strange for them too, but you need them. They are your emotional support system; they constantly reassure you of your value as a person, well or ill. Expressing your feelings by sharing them with other people takes the edge off the pain and puts things in perspective. It is good policy to talk to many people, rather than just one or two. This way there is no danger on the one hand of burdening any one person, or on the other of hurting someone's feelings— "Why didn't you tell me?"

People like to feel they can help—and anyone who can make you laugh is worth their weight in gold.

DEPRESSION AND ANXIETY

You are bound to feel unhappy and anxious some of the time. The understandable lowering of mood and haunting anxiety about the illness sometimes peaks into panicky feelings when a crisis threatens—how will you cope? When it actually happens, nine times out of ten you will rise to the occasion and do all the right things automatically. On the tenth time it will be taken out of your hands. The medics will know what to do.

Ralph

Ralph was a man who prided himself on never losing his cool. All through the ups and downs of his Crohn's over the last eight years, he had managed to keep his sense of control. He discussed his medication and the dosage with the doctor, and he understood his explanations of the pathology underlying the symptoms and what the barium enema showed. Ralph decided against having a colonoscopy, although the gastroenterologist advised it. Ralph's disease was mainly in the colon, and through care with his diet, regular prednisolone, and willpower, he had managed to take hardly any time off work.

"Better than the youngsters," he would boast. He was now 58. It happened in March, when he was taking a brisk walk in a biting east wind. His blood pressure, which had been creeping up over the last few years, must have reacted to the cold and the exercise with a sudden surge. Ralph noticed a weird, warm feeling of blood pouring from his anal passage. He had not the slightest control over it and he began to feel dizzy. He was frightened, a feeling he had never before admitted in himself, and was thankful to be bundled into an ambulance. From then until after the operation, he let other people take responsibility for decision making.

It took him two or three months to get the hang of the ileostomy but much longer to come to terms with having lost his colon. Now, 18 months later, Ralph is back in control of his body—including its changed anatomy—his feelings, and his job. He sees himself as something of an expert in Crohn's. The other bonus is that he and his wife have learned to talk about their feelings as well as the illness.

CLINICAL DEPRESSION

Mild anxiety and depression are endemic in Crohn's disease. Clinical depression and anxiety are something else. They are illnesses in their own right and require specialized treatment. Depression as an illness not only drains energy, it takes away hope and any possibility of happiness or of feeling anything at all for loved ones. Guilt takes over, not for anything the sufferer has done but just for being herself or himself. Even sleep brings no relief. Although the depression feels like a life sentence, one can emerge from this black hole—but treatment is essential to prevent its lingering for months.

Esther

Esther was devastated to find that she had Crohn's disease. Her boyfriend split when he felt she was being a drag, and this did not help, especially as she had argued with her parents over him. Esther was 17 and no more moody than most teenagers. Her mother had experienced mild postnatal depression after Esther was born, but otherwise there was no history of psychiatric illness in the family. Her parents were worried about the Crohn's, but not greatly concerned about her occasional depressed periods.

Esther had been put on a fairly high dose of prednisolone to control the pain and diarrhea initially, and this may have been partly responsible for the low, negative mood that now engulfed her. She would not eat, did not want to talk, and spent most of the day sitting and staring. She could not be bothered to put on any makeup or care what clothes she wore. She blamed herself for the illness—which was not at all like her. She felt worse as the days passed and went to bed early to escape her feelings, but she found she could not sleep.

Esther had clinical depression. The counselor affiliated with the clinic could do nothing to lift her mood. Esther needed the full antidepressant package, starting with seven weeks of intensive treatment with medication and cognitive therapy. She continued with the latter while the medication was reduced, but not stopped, for another five months, and she was able to go back to college partway through. Maintenance treatment with medicines and discussion sessions, first on a monthly basis, then two times a month, continued for the rest of the year. The Crohn's symptoms had also been brought under control, now with nonsteroid drugs. By the time Esther was through with the psychiatric treatment, like other sufferers from clinical depression, there had been plenty of opportunities to discuss and work through the stresses that had built up.

Cognitive psychotherapy is a talking treatment in which you are guided, logically, into understanding your mental state and getting rid of the harmful automatic thoughts and reactions that are maintaining the depression. Without medication such treatment can be effective for depression but may be expensive. Some insurance policies limit benefits for psychiatric/psychotherapy sessions. To avoid being caught unaware, check your insurance benefits carefully. As another option, some nonprofit organizations such as the United Way offer counseling or psychotherapy sessions on a sliding-scale basis. Many university clinics make such services available to students free or on a sliding scale.

ANXIETY

Anxiety is acutely distressing, but it usually does not carry the depressive guilt and hopelessness that can get so bad that suicide seems an option. Medication, including some of the modern, post-Prozac antidepressants, may also help in anxiety, but it is more a matter for constructive discussion with a psychologist, and active involvement in overcoming whatever you fear.

Both depression and anxiety are liable to recur if there is a sudden downturn in your physical state, or some other blow, or a slow buildup of stress—for instance at work. No one can keep stress out of their life long term. The trick is to manage it.

One big stressful event is having an operation involving a colostomy or ileostomy. This is a major life change, and you must allow time for your body, and even more important, your mind, to adjust, for there to be harmonious cooperation between the two. The practical aspects are dealt with in chapter 10, but being at peace with yourself with a changed body can be hard to achieve. A firm foundation lies in building good relationships—at home, in the outside world, at work. If they were less than satisfactory before, now is an opportunity, as a new, mended person, to put that right.

People are your lifeline, even when your anxiety or depressed mood tells you to shut yourself away. Time on your own—to think too much—is bad for you, and although you need adequate sleep (six to eight hours) too much time in bed will lower your mood. Since your stoma is now part of you, you may as well start living to your full potential with it. Of course there will be days when you have had it, and feel down or worried, but live through these, pick yourself up, and carry on. This is the achievement to be proud of.

While depression and anxiety can be disabling illnesses in themselves, often they accompany having Crohn's. You need to evolve ways to protect yourself against them. Here are some techniques that work for me:

- Keeping friendships in good repair.

- Sharing your feelings and ideas when they are fresh, not only with established friends but new acquaintances, too. Not everybody will want to know the physical details about your bowels, but they can all relate to feelings of worry or sadness—or what you look forward to or hope for. Day-to-day conversation is safer and better than popping Valium, and it relaxes your mind and body just as effectively.

- Exercise, which can both stimulate and relax, whether it is a session in the gym or pool, or simply a half-hour walk.

- Exchanging affection with a dog or a cat. Contact with pets is known to boost the immune system and promote healing, but better still must be sharing feelings with your loved ones.

Chapter 15

The Research Continues

Richard Quain, writing on chronic inflammation of the intestines in 1885, remarked what a "debilitating and wearying" condition it was—and, at that time, invariably fatal. The methods of examination when the abdomen was "the seat of the mischief" were simple:

- Inspection of the size and shape of the abdomen.

- Inserting a finger into the anal passage, or blowing air into it, though for what purpose is unclear.

- Examination of the stool with the naked eye.

Treatment was similarly limited:

- quinine

- iron

- sea air

- removal of mental worry

Fifty years later Burrill Crohn suggested that "his" disease might be caused by some species of mycobacterium, similar to the one responsible for tuberculosis. Research into Crohn's disease ran round in circles for another half century, vainly trying to find the bug. Meanwhile DNA was discovered and we had entered the technological age.

In 1989 Professor Joseph Kirsner of Chicago was confidently forecasting the use of DNA probes to identify different species of microorganisms, although he was bemoaning the lack of success in linking any one of them convincingly with Crohn's. The disease was already becoming more common (current estimates suggest up to one million cases exist in the United States) and although the areas most affected were in Western Europe and North America, it appeared to have a worldwide distribution. Kirsner knew of cases in Algeria, Bagwanath, and among the Chinese in Canada. He thought that autoimmunity was a key cause, possibly through proteins from viruses or bacteria becoming incorporated into the lining cells of the gut. He had hopes of a vaccine being developed against all autoimmune disease. This has not yet happened.

The mechanism by which stress is implicated in Crohn's in both humans and cows still needs investigating, and also how smoking fits in. Pharmaceutical research has produced ever more effective medicines—each with its potential for side effects. Cyclosporine, used in difficult cases of Crohn's, is one such. The first report of serious effects on the brain and nervous system with this drug came out in the *British Medical Journal* in April 1999. It seems that the danger occurs when cyclosporine is used in conjunction with some other medicines, including prednisolone and methotrexate. The first is used frequently in Crohn's, the latter occasionally.

On the surgical front, stricturoplasty, a simple, localized operation, has become the standard for relieving intestinal obstruction or the threat of it, and microsurgical instruments are constantly being improved. Another advance is in cancer surveillance. Cancer is a complication that can arise in long-term Crohn's disease. There are now techniques for detecting the early, precancerous changes before an actual cancer develops, in the same way as a cervical smear.

In the early 1990s, Professor J. Hermon-Taylor and his team from St. George's Hospital, London, entered the arena with outstanding zeal for their mycobacterium theory of the cause of Crohn's. Since 1913, even before Crohn published his work, something akin to Mycobacterium tuberculosis was suspected of being responsible for inflammation of the intestines in humans as well as cows. They could not see it, but they called it Mycobacterium paratuberculosis (Mptb). We now believe that this bug can live in the soil, in rivers, and on plants, and that cows can harbor Mptb without being ill. Some of them, however, develop a Crohn's-like illness, Johne's disease. Modern, intensive milk-production methods may serve to concentrate these bacteria in certain places.

Two major problems affecting research have been, first, the difficulty in identifying Mptb from the many other microorganisms in cattle and human feces, and second, growing it in culture. Now the polymerase chain reaction (PCR) in combination with increasingly refined DNA probes can identify Mptb, even in small quantities, though not yet as a routine procedure. A tiresome stumbling block remains: the fastidious nature of Mptb, which takes many months to grow in culture, if at all.

Food scares are commonplace, and Mptb has provided two. In 1996 Professor Hermon-Taylor suggested that Mptb in milk and milk products could infect people and cause Crohn's disease. Nothing much was done about this. More recently, he indicated that drinking water might also be a vehicle for Mptb. Cattle slurry could possibly be contaminating water supplies. This view was aired on British television news in April 1999. Apparently some of these bacteria can survive pasteurization, in the case of milk, and the water-purification process. This, of course, does not prove that taking in some Mptb causes Crohn's in normal circumstances. We all swallow millions of germs in our daily lives.

However, one study shows that more people with Crohn's have Mptb in their intestines than those without Crohn's, including sufferers from ulcerative colitis, which Crohn's so much resembles. If Mptb is a major cause of Crohn's disease, it should be curable with antimycobacterial antibiotics, such as azithromycin or clarithromycin. These and other drugs are currently the subject of trials, but there has been no breakthrough. Any beneficial effects have been slow to develop and have not been dramatic.

Professor Hermon-Taylor's theories are attractive, and it may well be that Mptb is heavily implicated in a fair proportion of cases, but it cannot be the sole cause of the disease. The connection with ulcerative colitis, including what appears to be a genetic link, yet the marked differences between the two illnesses, remains unexplained. Or why one is more likely to develop Crohn's if one has a brother or sister with the disease than a parent.

Those who work in the field of Crohn's and know most about it, are divided over Professor Hermon-Taylor's ideas. The National Association for Colitis and Crohn's disease (NACC), in the U.K., is highly skeptical. The good thing is that the British government has now pledged to investigate the whole matter "extremely seriously."

What causes Crohn's disease? Perhaps we will find the answer, and perhaps that answer will lead to healthy prevention or a cure. Until then, Crohn's patients have the benefits of modern medical and surgical techniques and dietary knowledge—all of which continue to advance regularly—on their side. Unlike a few generations ago, today it is possible to live with a chronic disorder such as Crohn's and still enjoy a full life. What is required is becoming educated about the positive options available, deciding with the help of health-care professionals which courses of action will work best for you, making use of your support system of friends and loved ones, and remaining flexible and open to new treatments. Last but not least, as in treating any illness, maintaining a healthy, realistic sense of optimism may be most important of all.

Resources

UNITED STATES

Crohn's and Colitis Foundation of America, Inc. (CCFA)
386 Park Avenue South, 17th Floor
New York, NY 10016-8804
Tel.: 212-685-3440; toll free 800-932-2423
E-mail: info@ccfa.org
http://www.ccfa.org/

Crohn's Disease Resource Center Web Site (links page)
http://www.healingwell.com/ibd
Intestinal Disease Foundation
1323 Forbes Avenue, Suite 200
Pittsburgh, PA 15219
Tel.: 412-261-5888

National Digestive Diseases Information Clearinghouse (NDDIC)
A service of the National Institute of Diabetes and Digestive and Kidney Diseases (NIDDK), which is part of the federal-government-sponsored National Institutes of Health (NIH).

2 Information Way
Bethesda, MD 20892-3570
Tel.: 301-654-3810

E-mail: nddic@info.niddk.nih.gov
http://www.niddk.nih.gov/health/digest/pubs/crohns/crohns.htm

Pediatric Crohn's and Colitis Association, Inc.
P.O. Box 188
Newton, MA 02468
Tel.: 617-489-5854
E-mail: questions@pcca.hypermart.net
http://pcca.hypermart.net

United Ostomy Association, Inc.
19772 MacArthur Blvd., Suite 200
Irvine, CA 92612-2405
Tel.: 949-660-8624; toll free 800-826-0826
Fax: 949-660-9262
E-mail: uoa@deltanet.com
http://www.uoa.org

CANADA

Crohn's and Colitis Foundation of Canada (CCFC)
21 St. Clair Avenue East, Suite 301
Toronto, Ontario
Canada M4T 1L9
Tel.: 416-920-5035; toll free: 800-387-1479
Fax: 416-929-0364
http://www.ccfc.ca

UNITED KINGDOM

National Association for Colitis and Crohn's Disease (NACC)
P.O. Box 205
St. Albans, Herts AL1 5HH
U.K.
Tel.: +44 01727 844296
http://www.nacc.org.uk/contact.htm

Crohn's in Childhood Research Association (CICRA)
356 West Barnes Lane
Motspur Park, Surrey KT3 6NB
U.K.
Tel.: +44 0208 949 6209

Teens with Crohn's Disease Web Site
http://pages.prodigy.com/teencron/

British Colostomy Association
15 Station Road
Reading, Berks RG1 1LG
U.K.
Tel. (toll free from inside U.K.): 0800 328 4257

The Ileostomy and Internal Pouch Support Group
P.O. Box 123
Scunthorpe, North Lincs DN15 9YW
U.K.
Tel.: +44 01724 844296
http://www.ileostomypouch.demon.co.uk

National Ankylosing Spondylitis Society (NASS)
P.O. Box 179
Mayfield, East Sussex TN40 6ZL
U.K.
Tel.: +44 01435 873527
http://web.ukonline.co.uk/nass/

EUROPE

**European Foundation of Crohn's and Ulcerative Colitis
Associations (EFFCA)**
Eighteen associations throughout Europe
Secretariat: Beukenlaan 3
4356 HJ Oostkapelle
The Netherlands
Tel.: +31 (0) 118 58 60 73
http://www.nacc.org.uk/effca/efcmem.htm

AUSTRALIA AND NEW ZEALAND

Australian Crohn's and Colitis Association Inc. (ACCA)
P.O. Box 201
Mooroolbark, Victoria 3138
Australia
Tel.: +61 3 9276 9914
E-mail: acca@ozramp.net.au

Australian Crohn's and Colitis Association (Qld) Inc (ACCAQ)
P.O. Box 548
Maleny, Queensland 4552
Australia
Tel.: +61 7 5494 2149
http://www.accaq.org.au

South Australia Crohn's and Colitis Association Inc. (SACCA)
P.O. Box 3153
Rundle Mail, Adelaide, SA 5000
Australia
Tel.: +61 8 8449 4357
http://www.accaq.org.au/text/affiliates/acca.htm

Crohn's and Colitis Support Group Inc (CCSG)
P.O. Box 24-171
Royal Oak, Auckland
New Zealand
Tel.: +64 9 6367228
http://home.clear.net.nz/pages/ccsg/clearhome.html

Index

FAD-FREE NUTRITION *by* Fredrick J. Stare, M.D., Ph.D., and Elizabeth M. Whelan, Sc.D., M.P.H.

From the American Council on Science and Health, a no-nonsense book about how to enjoy the pleasures of eating again.... Forget the trendy diets and weight the facts—this book offers sound information about how to get back to the simplicity of eating. From explaining why the produce at the supermarket is indeed safe to describing which foods can boost immune systems to showing how easy the food pyramid really is, this book takes the fright out of food.

256 pages ... Paperback ... $14.95

GET FIT WHILE YOU SIT: Easy Workouts from Your Chair *by* Charlene Torkelson

Here is a total body workout that can be done right from your chair, anywhere. It is perfect for office workers, travelers, and those with age-related movement limitations or special conditions. The book offers three programs. The One-Hour Chair Program is a full-body, low-impact workout that includes light aerobics and exercises to be done with or without weights. The 5-Day Short Program features five compact workouts for those short on time. Finally, the Ten-Minute Miracles is a group of easy-to-do exercises perfect for anyone on the go.

160 pages ... 212 b/w photos ... Paperback $12.95 ... Hard Cover $22.95

ALTERNATIVE TREATMENTS FOR FIBROMYALGIA AND CHRONIC FATIGUE SYNDROME: Insights from Practitioners and Patients *by* Mari Skelly and Andrea Helm, Foreword by Paul Brown, M.D., Ph.D.

If you or someone you love suffers from FM and CFS, you know that conventional medicine may not always help. This book describes a wide range of alternative therapies from acupuncture to massage to yoga and more. It includes interviews with treatment professionals and personal stories from sufferers, who describe the individual drug, diet and activity regimens that help them. Information on legal issues, such as obtaining Social Security disability, and a comprehensive resource section are also included.

288 pages ... Paperback $15.95 ... Hard Cover $25.95

To order books see last page or call (800) 266-5592

ONCE A MONTH: Understanding and Treating PMS

by Katharina Dalton, M.D. Revised 6th edition

Once considered an imaginary complaint, PMS has at last received the serious attention it deserves, thanks largely to the work of Katharina Dalton, M.D. Fully one-third of the material is new in this sixth edition, from the latest research on how PMS affects learning to the PMS/menopause connection. Most importantly, Dr. Dalton addresses the whole range of possible treatments—from self-care methods such as the three-hourly starch diet and relaxation techniques to the newest medical options, including updated guidelines for progesterone therapy.

320 pages ... 55 illus. ... Paperback $15.95

ANDROGEN DISORDERS IN WOMEN: The Most Neglected Hormone Problem by Theresa Cheung

One in ten women in the U.S. suffers from a disorder caused by an imbalance of the so-called "male hormones" known as androgens. Symptoms may include facial or body hair growth or loss, dull skin, fatigue, and weight gain. Because doctors tend to dismiss or ignore such symptoms, there has been little information available on androgen disorders—until now. This book discusses the medical and emotional effects that excessive androgens can have, and outlines the various forms of conventional and alternative treatment.

224 pages ... Paperback $13.95 ... Hard cover $23.95

HER HEALTHY HEART: A Woman's Guide to Preventing and Reversing Heart Disease Naturally

by Linda Ojeda, Ph.D.

Heart disease is the #1 killer of American women ages 44 to 65, yet most of the research is done on men. HER HEALTHY HEART fills this gap by addressing the unique aspects of heart disease in women and natural ways to combat it. Dr. Ojeda explains how women can prevent heart disease whether they take hormone replacement therapy (HRT) or not. She also provides information on how women can reduce their risk of heart disease by making changes in diet, increasing physical activity, and managing stress. A 50-item lifestyle questionnaire helps women discover areas to work on.

352 pages ... 7 illus. ... Paperback $14.95 ... Hard cover $24.95

To order books see last page or call (800) 266-5592

CANCER—INCREASING YOUR ODDS FOR SURVIVAL: A Resource Guide for Integrating Mainstream, Alternative and Complementary Therapies *by* David Bognar

Based on the four-part television series hosted by Walter Cronkite, this book provides a comprehensive look at traditional medical treatments for cancer and how these can be supplemented. It explains the basics of cancer and the best actions to take immediately after a diagnosis of cancer. It outlines the various conventional, alternative, and complementary treatments; describes the powerful effect the mind can have on the body and the therapies that strengthen this connection; and explores spiritual healing and issues surrounding death and dying. Includes full-length interviews with leaders in the field of healing, including Joan Borysenko, Stephen Levine, and Bernie Siegel.

352 pages ... Paperback $15.95 ... Hard cover $25.95

WOMEN'S CANCERS: How to Prevent Them, How to Treat Them, How to Beat Them

by Kerry A. McGinn, R.N. and Pamela J. Haylock, R.N.

WOMEN'S CANCERS is the first book to focus specifically on the cancers that affect only women—breast, cervical, ovarian, and uterine. It offers the latest information in a clear style and discusses all the issues, from the psychological to the practical, surrounding a cancer diagnosis.

"WOMEN'S CANCERS is fully comprehensive, helpful to patients and healthcare workers alike. Recommended." —LIBRARY JOURNAL

512 pages ... 68 illus. ... 2nd edition ... Paperback $19.95 ... Hardcover $29.95

THE FEISTY WOMAN'S BREAST CANCER BOOK

by Elaine Ratner. Featured in *The New York Times*

This personal, advice-packed guide helps women navigate the emotional and psychological landscape surrounding breast cancer, and make their own decisions with confidence. Its insight and positive message make this a perfect companion for every feisty woman who wants not only to survive but thrive after breast cancer.

"There are times when a woman needs a wise and level-headed friend, someone kind, savvy and, and caring...[This] book...is just such a friend..." —Rachel Naomi Remen, M.D., author of *Kitchen Table Wisdom*

288 pages ... Paperback $14.95 ... Hardcover $24.95

To order books see last page or call (800) 266-5592

ORDER FORM

10% DISCOUNT on orders of $50 or more —
20% DISCOUNT on orders of $150 or more —
30% DISCOUNT on orders of $500 or more —
On cost of books for fully prepaid orders

NAME

ADDRESS

CITY/STATE   ZIP/POSTCODE

PHONE   COUNTRY (outside of U.S.)

TITLE	QTY	PRICE	TOTAL
Positive Options for Crohn's...(paperback)		@ $12.95	
Positive Options for Crohn's...(hardcover)		@ $22.95	

Prices subject to change without notice

Please list other titles below:

		@ $	
		@ $	
		@ $	
		@ $	
		@ $	
		@ $	
		@ $	

Check here to receive our book catalog ❑   FREE

Shipping Costs:
First book: $3.00 by book post ($4.50 by UPS, Priority Mail, or to ship outside the U.S.)
Each additional book: $1.00
For rush orders and bulk shipments call us at (800) 266-5592

TOTAL _____
Less discount @____% (_____)
TOTAL COST OF BOOKS _____
Calif. residents add sales tax _____
Shipping & handling _____
TOTAL ENCLOSED _____
Please pay in U.S. funds only

❑ Check ❑ Money Order ❑ Visa ❑ Mastercard ❑ Discover

Card # _____ Exp. date _____

Signature _____

Complete and mail to:
Hunter House Inc., Publishers
PO Box 2914, Alameda CA 94501-0914
Orders: (800) 266-5592   email: ordering@hunterhouse.com
Phone (510) 865-5282 Fax (510) 865-4295
❑ Check here to receive our book catalog

POC 12/03